Waltham Forest Libraries

Please return this item by the last date stamped. The loan may be renewed unless required by another customer.

01/18		

Need to renew your books?
http://www.walthamforest.gov.uk/libraries or
Dial 0333 370 4700 for Callpoint – our 24/7 automated telephone renewal line. You will need your library card number and PIN. If you do not know your PIN, contact your local library

Substantial discounts on bulk quantities of Summersdale books are available to corporations, professional associations and other organisations. For details contact general enquiries: telephone: +44 (0) 1243 771107 or email: enquiries@summersdale.com.

PREGNANCY
MADE SIMPLE

AN ILLUSTRATED GUIDE
FROM CONCEPTION
TO BIRTH

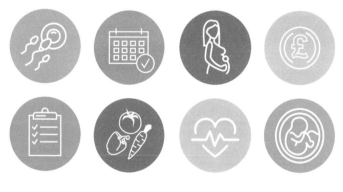

Claire Plimmer

DISCLAIMER

No two pregnancies are the same, because every woman is unique. The information and advice provided in this book is of a general nature, and therefore it may not be applicable in all instances.

Every effort has been made to ensure that the information in this book is accurate and current at the time of publication. The author and the publisher cannot accept responsibility for any misuse or misunderstanding of any information contained herein, or any loss, damage or injury, be it health, financial or otherwise, suffered by any individual or group acting upon or relying on information contained herein.

None of the opinions or suggestions in this book is intended to replace medical opinion. If you have concerns about your, or your baby's health, please seek professional advice.

CONTENTS

CHAPTER 4: WELL-BEING...101

CHAPTER 5: FINAL STAGES..138

INTRODUCTION

Pregnancy can sometimes seem like an overwhelming subject for parents-to-be. But fear not. The following chapters will take you through this amazing journey, from beginning to end, in a fresh, simple and helpful way.

Each chapter has been designed to give you a balance of essential advice and fascinating trivia. From the basics of fertility and conception through to the miracle of giving birth, this colourful and creative book will be your trusty companion, based on up-to-date information and the experience of real women.

Whether you're a first-time mother, a curious dad, or just looking to offer informed advice and support, you'll find plenty of useful tips and intriguing facts in the pages that follow.

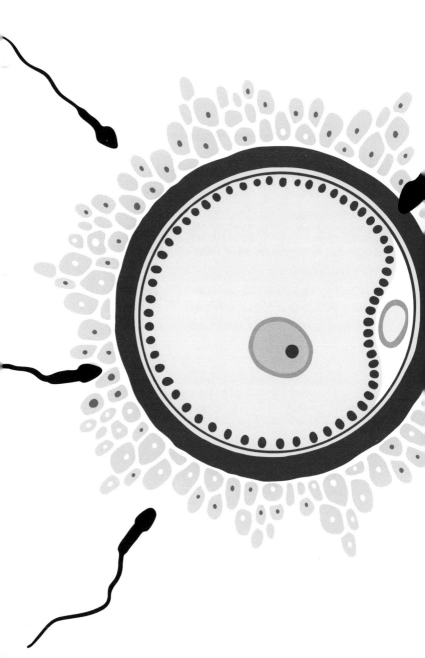

CHAPTER 1

GETTING PREGNANT

INTRODUCTION

The decision to have a baby is life-changing. Some couples may find themselves pregnant after the first attempt at conceiving, while others will struggle for many years. In order to give you the best chance at successfully starting the journey towards parenthood, there are many lifestyle changes you can make. This chapter is a guide to all the things you can do, both individually and as a couple, in order to maximise your fertility and thereby maximise your chance of conception and a healthy pregnancy.

CONCEPTION FACTS: EGGS

By her twelfth week in the womb, a female foetus will have produced all the eggs she will ever carry in her lifetime. These undeveloped eggs will lie dormant within her ovaries until she reaches puberty, when they will begin to be released (usually once a month) from a follicle into the fallopian tube.

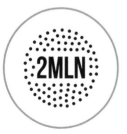

Women are born with all the eggs they'll have in their lifetime (around 2 million). Which means, effectively, that your maternal grandmother carried you as an unfertilised egg when she was about to give birth to your mother.

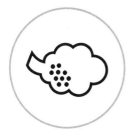

But by the time a woman reaches puberty, only about 300,000 to 400,000 eggs are left. Around 1,000 will die during each menstrual cycle. A woman at the age of 40 will have only about 60,000 eggs.

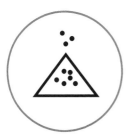

Around 400–500 mature eggs are released from the ovaries in a typical woman's lifetime.

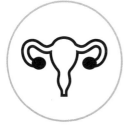

An egg is the size of a grain of sand (around 0.12 mm / 0.005 inches), which is visible to the naked eye.

The matured egg only lives about 12 to 24 hours before being expelled during menstruation.

CONCEPTION FACTS: SPERM

Over the course of his lifetime, a man will produce around 525 billion sperm, and will ejaculate around a billion sperm every month (depending on how sexually active he is). Each ejaculation contains around 3 ml / 0.1 fl oz of semen, which contains around 100 million sperm. Of these, only 1 in 14 million will actually reach the fallopian tube – most die in the journey from the cervix. And only a single sperm can fulfil its ultimate purpose of fertilising the egg.

- At the moment of fertilisation, the tail of the sperm breaks off and only the head will penetrate the egg. It does this by producing an enzyme called acrosome to dissolve the outer layer of the egg.

- Each sperm has a unique genetic code. It contains the 23 chromosomes that will combine with the mother's to create a zygote (fertilised egg) with 46 chromosomes. The combination of these chromosomes is random and unique.

- As soon as one sperm penetrates the egg (or ovum), the egg secretes a membrane to prevent any other sperm getting in.

- Sperm can live for up to five days inside the uterus, meaning conception can happen several days after sexual intercourse.

WHAT MAKES A HEALTHY SPERM?

 TIMING

The frequency of ejaculation will affect a man's sperm count. Too much ejaculation means sperm production in the testes cannot keep up – therefore, having more sex does not necessarily increase your chances of conceiving.

 DIET

A man's diet is very important. Foods that contain high levels of selenium, zinc and Vitamin D will improve sperm motility (the ability to swim towards the egg). Antioxidant-rich foods such as fruit will also help improve the quality of the sperm.

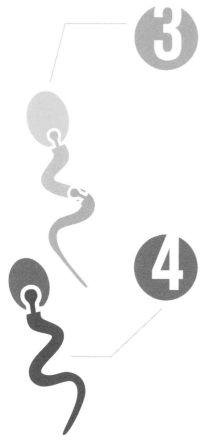

3 AGE

Although men can father a child into their seventies and beyond, the older the man, the longer it will take to conceive. Men are 92 per cent likely to conceive within a year if they are under 25, whereas only 85 per cent of men over 35 will manage conception in under a year. This percentage steadily declines as age increases.

4 FITNESS

The sperm of a smoker or a heavy drinker will have significantly less motility than that of a healthy man. Being obese can also significantly reduce the quality and quantity of sperm as well as affecting the ability to get an erection.

CONCEPTION STATISTICS

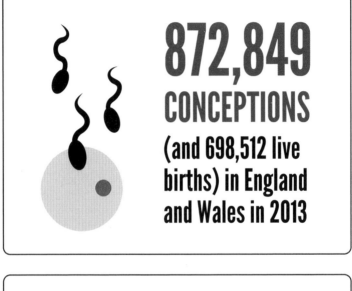

872,849 CONCEPTIONS (and 698,512 live births) in England and Wales in 2013

1 IN 7 COUPLES may have difficulty conceiving

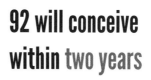

FOR EVERY 100 COUPLES TRYING TO CONCEIVE NATURALLY:

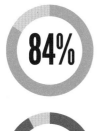

84 will conceive within one year

92 will conceive within two years

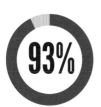

93 will conceive within three years

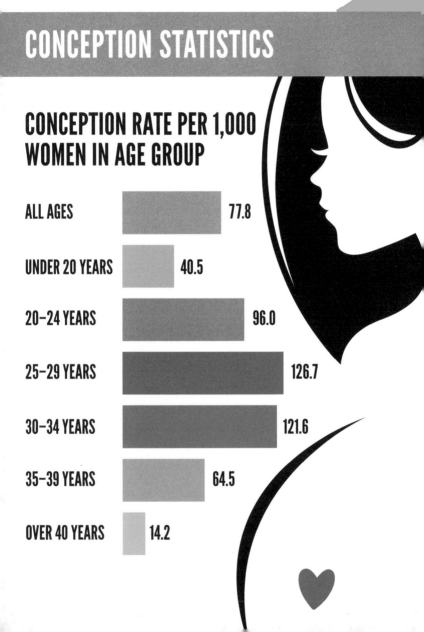

CONCEPTION STATISTICS

CONCEPTION RATE PER 1,000 WOMEN IN AGE GROUP

ALL AGES	77.8
UNDER 20 YEARS	40.5
20–24 YEARS	96.0
25–29 YEARS	126.7
30–34 YEARS	121.6
35–39 YEARS	64.5
OVER 40 YEARS	14.2

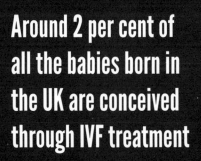

Around 2 per cent of all the babies born in the UK are conceived through IVF treatment

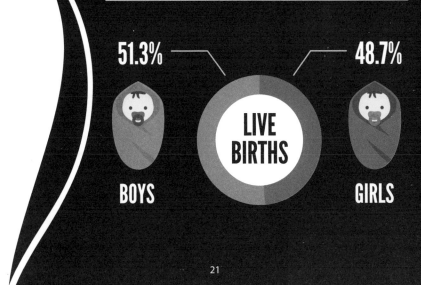

51.3%

48.7%

LIVE BIRTHS

BOYS

GIRLS

FERTILITY ISSUES: INFERTILITY

The World Health Organization (WHO) defines infertility as a failure to conceive after 12 months of having sex without using any form of contraception. This definition includes either being unable to conceive at all, or not being able to maintain a pregnancy once it has begun. There are many causes of infertility, in both men and women, but having any of the following problems does not always result in an inability to become pregnant. You should always discuss any concerns or symptoms with your doctor.

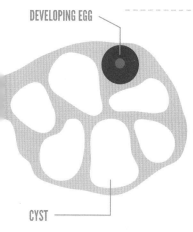

DEVELOPING EGG

CYST

POLYCYSTIC OVARY SYNDROME (PCOS)

How common?
Perhaps as many as 1 in 10 women of childbearing age.

This hormonal condition – in which cysts develop in the ovaries and disrupt regular ovulation – can be characterised by symptoms such as irregular or no periods, pelvic pain, and excess hair on the face or body.

ENDOMETRIOSIS

How common?   Possibly also 1 in 10 women of childbearing age.

This is a condition where small pieces of the womb lining, known as the endometrium, start growing in other places, such as the ovaries, causing pelvic pain and infertility.

PELVIC INFLAMMATORY DISEASE (PID)

How common? **Very common, but it's difficult to estimate exact prevalence – 1 in 4 cases are known to be the result of a sexually transmitted infection (STI).**

PID happens when bacteria cause an infection and swelling in the uterus and fallopian tubes. It can also lead to an increase in the likelihood of an ectopic pregnancy.

EMBRYO

ECTOPIC PREGNANCY

How common?
Around 1 in every 100 pregnancies.

An ectopic pregnancy happens when a fertilised egg implants itself outside the womb, usually in a fallopian tube. This can result in damage to the fallopian tube and can cause life-threatening bleeding. Signs of a ruptured fallopian tube are severe, acute pain, dizziness, sickness and diarrhoea. If you think this is happening to you, seek immediate medical attention.

LOW SPERM COUNT

How common? **Up to 1 in 5 men aged 18–25 have a low sperm count, defined as fewer than 20 million sperm per millilitre of semen.**

Infertility may be the result of low sperm count or low sperm motility, where the sperm he produces are not strong enough swimmers to fertilise an egg. Genetic or environmental factors may also lead to sperm abnormalities that may affect fertility. See pages 28–9 for tips on how to improve sperm quantity and quality.

FERTILITY ISSUES:
SOLUTIONS FOR INFERTILITY

Depending on the reason
for infertility, there are
many solutions to the
problem, including
artificial insemination,
IVF and genetic
testing. Many people
also find alternative
therapies such as
acupuncture helpful.

FERTILITY ISSUES: IVF FACTS

The techniques behind in-vitro fertilisation (IVF) have been developing since the first 'test-tube' baby, Louise Brown, was born in the UK in 1978. IVF is considered a 'last resort' treatment as it is both costly and physically demanding on the woman.

 AROUND 50,000 WOMEN ATTEMPT TO CONCEIVE THROUGH IVF ANNUALLY IN THE UK, AND THIS FIGURE IS RISING EVERY YEAR

 AROUND 15 EGGS ARE EXTRACTED FROM THE OVARIES

 EACH CYCLE OF TREATMENT HAS ABOUT A 25% CHANCE OF A SUCCESSFUL BIRTH

 THE AVERAGE AGE FOR A WOMAN'S FIRST CYCLE OF IVF TREATMENT IS 35

FERTILITY ISSUES: MISCARRIAGE

Defined as the loss of pregnancy during the first 23 weeks, miscarriage can happen to every woman and, in fact, over half of early pregnancies end in a miscarriage, but these are often undetected. The vast majority of women go on to have a successful pregnancy. The fertilised egg may not become a viable pregnancy for many reasons, including:

- a failed implantation of the egg

- low levels of the hormone progesterone in the woman

- genetic abnormalities in the fertilised egg

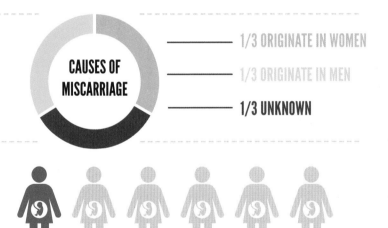

CAUSES OF MISCARRIAGE

——————— 1/3 ORIGINATE IN WOMEN

——————— 1/3 ORIGINATE IN MEN

——————— 1/3 UNKNOWN

Estimated frequency of miscarriage: 1 in 6 women
Estimated frequency of recurrent miscarriage (three or more consecutive miscarriages): 1 in 100 women

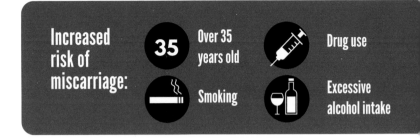

Increased risk of miscarriage:

35 Over 35 years old

Drug use

Smoking

Excessive alcohol intake

COPING WITH MISCARRIAGE

Although most pregnancies result in a happy, healthy baby, sadly there are some instances when this doesn't happen. If you're unlucky enough to lose your baby during any stage of your pregnancy, or have a stillbirth, it's important that you and your family have the support you need in this devastating time. If you have a later miscarriage, you can choose to have a memorial, burial or cremation. Stillbirths must be formally registered but this is not required with a miscarriage. Some hospitals can provide a certificate if you wish. Your doctor should be able to guide you and arrange bereavement counselling, if you feel that it would help. There's no doubt that suffering a miscarriage or stillbirth is a horrendous experience. You may feel as though you'll never recover, emotionally. But take heart and remember that it does not affect your chances of becoming pregnant again and going on to have a healthy baby in the future.

BOOST YOUR CHANCES: WHAT CAN MEN DO?

Men can make a number of changes in their everyday lives to aid their fertility, boost their sperm count and sperm motility, giving themselves the best chance of successfully fathering healthy children.

1 Consider your job – try to make adjustments if your work involves exposure to harsh chemicals such as fertilisers. Some studies have found that regular contact with chemicals can affect motility and increase the risk of sperm abnormalities

2 Eat a healthy, balanced diet, rich in whole and unprocessed foods – this will provide your body with vitamins and minerals, notably zinc, which are essential for the production of healthy sperm

3 Take regular exercise – as well as the proven benefits of exercise for overall health and reducing stress, this will increase your body's levels of the hormone testosterone, which will give your libido a helpful boost

4 Aim to ejaculate every other day – every day would mean testicles would struggle to keep up with production

5 Make changes as early as possible – sperm production takes a while (typically 64 days until maturation) so sooner is better to allow the changes to take effect

BOOST YOUR CHANCES: WHAT SHOULD MEN AVOID?

 Avoid too much exposure to heat, **including laptops and hot baths, to regulate the temperature of your testicles**

 Stop smoking, **as it has an adverse effect on your sperm count and it has been shown to damage the membrane around the sperm**

 Avoid too-tight underwear **to allow air to circulate around your testicles**

 Reduce your consumption of alcohol – **drinking to excess can reduce sperm production and your body's testosterone levels**

 Avoid drugs and junk food – **these can affect your libido and ability to get an erection**

 Drink bottled water in preference to tap water – **some studies suggest that traces of the hormone oestrogen in tap water could adversely affect male fertility**

 Avoid stressful situations – **stress can lead to erectile dysfunction and may affect the quality of your sperm**

WHAT YOU CAN DO WITH YOUR PARTNER

To strengthen your bond as a couple, leading to
greater intimacy and a healthier relationship,
try any or all of the following ideas.

- **Make sure you spend quality time together that doesn't revolve around trying to conceive. It might be a short trip to the local park, or perhaps a holiday overseas.**

- **Learn how to perform a proper massage and practise on each other to encourage relaxation and increase intimacy.**

- **Start a home-decorating project to feel like you are really getting ready for your new arrival.**

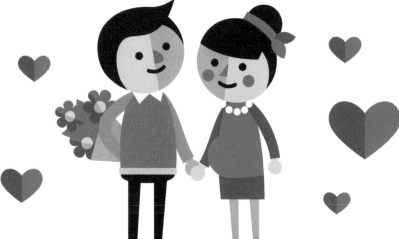

BOOST YOUR CHANCES: SEX

Statistics show that, up to a point, the more frequent the sex between partners (as opposed to masturbation), the less time it takes to conceive in the long term. If you have sex every day, however, a man's testicles may struggle to keep up with sperm production, so sex every other day is better.

Once a month	**43 months**
3 times a month	**15 months**
10 times a month	**5 months**
15+ times a month	**3.5 months**

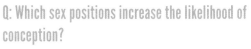

SEX FAQ

Q: Which sex positions increase the likelihood of conception?

A: All of them. There's no proof that any one is better than another.

Q: Will having sex in a certain position help me have a boy/girl?

A: No. There are plenty of theories, but none have been proven.

Q: Should I stay lying down afterwards?

A: It's worth a try, as it may help the sperm enter your uterus and fallopian tubes.

GENERAL HEALTH

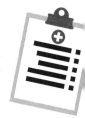

Good overall health makes getting pregnant simpler and safer, and it will give you peace of mind to know your body is in the best condition to produce and nurture a baby.

Go for a dental check-up prior to conception if possible – get all fillings done to avoid needing treatment (and x-rays) when pregnant.

Go for a medical check-up – ensure any long-term medication that you're taking is compatible with pregnancy.

Teeth are more vulnerable when you're pregnant due to hormonal changes, so making sure your dental health is in the best possible shape before you try for a baby is a good idea.

Check that you have immunity to major diseases, notably rubella as contracting it during pregnancy can have very serious consequences. Get any essential vaccinations.

SEXUAL HEALTH

Depending on your sexual history, it is worth being screened for sexually transmitted infections (STIs) as they can affect both your ability to conceive and the health of a developing foetus. It is also very important for men to be free from STIs if they are trying to conceive. Both sexes should get checked out for the following:

BACTERIAL INFECTIONS

Chlamydia – often symptomless, it can cause sterility in men and women if left untreated

Gonorrhea – frequently symptomless, untreated gonorrhea can cause pelvic inflammatory disease (PID) in women, which can lead to chronic pelvic pain, infertility and ectopic pregnancy

Syphilis – untreated syphilis can cause potentially life-threatening complications, and permanent damage to the brain, heart, bones and blood vessels. Pregnant women can pass syphilis on to their unborn children

VIRAL INFECTIONS

Herpes – the herpes simplex virus can infect oral or genital regions and may be passed by pregnant women to their babies during birth, causing possibly life-threatening complications of the central nervous system

Human immunodeficiency virus (HIV) – mothers may infect their babies during birth or through infected breast milk

Human papillomavirus (HPV) – can cause genital warts, which may present problems during pregnancy, including difficult urination and reduced elasticity of the vagina during delivery

BOOST YOUR CHANCES:
EXERCISE

 Both women and men, whether trying to conceive or not, should aim to do around 30 minutes of moderate exercise at least five days a week.

 You can also use the 'talk test' where an exercise is considered moderate if you can carry on a conversation while exercising. If you have difficulty speaking, then you are working too hard.

The best moderate exercise is walking. But yoga or Pilates are both excellent choices for women trying to conceive, due to their low impact.

Moderate exercise is any activity that gets your heart rate to 50–70 per cent of its maximum. Maximum heart rate is calculated by subtracting your age from 220.

STAY HYDRATED

It is important to stay hydrated throughout the day, but especially when doing exercise.

Recommended daily intake of water

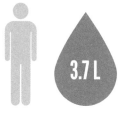 **3.7 L**

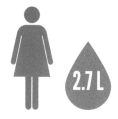 **2.7 L**

3.7 litres / 6.5 pints for a man | 2.7 litres / 4.75 pints for a woman

Water intake includes:

Water present in most food

Hot drinks

Tap and bottled water

BODY MASS INDEX

Apart from the enormous benefits of feeling healthy and full of energy, being fit and a sensible weight puts you at an advantage in terms of fertility. A good way to find out if you are the right weight for your size is to calculate your body mass index (BMI).

- To calculate your BMI, divide your weight in kilograms by your height in centimetres (or your weight in pounds by your height in feet)

- A healthy BMI is between 18.5 and 25

- For every BMI point above 29, women were 4 per cent less likely to conceive within a year

- If a woman's BMI is between 35 and 40, she is 43 per cent less likely to conceive within a year than if her BMI were 21

- Being overweight hinders fertility in several ways, including limiting the production of hormones called androgens, which in turn affects a woman's ability to produce oestrogen

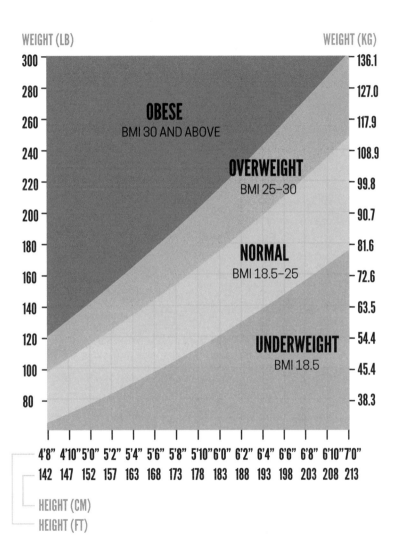

WEIGHT (LB)

WEIGHT (KG)

300 — — 136.1
280 — — 127.0
260 — — 117.9
240 — — 108.9
220 — — 99.8
200 — — 90.7
180 — — 81.6
160 — — 72.6
140 — — 63.5
120 — — 54.4
100 — — 45.4
80 — — 38.3

OBESE
BMI 30 AND ABOVE

OVERWEIGHT
BMI 25–30

NORMAL
BMI 18.5–25

UNDERWEIGHT
BMI 18.5

4'8" 4'10" 5'0" 5'2" 5'4" 5'6" 5'8" 5'10" 6'0" 6'2" 6'4" 6'6" 6'8" 6'10" 7'0"

142 147 152 157 163 168 173 178 183 188 193 198 203 208 213

HEIGHT (CM)
HEIGHT (FT)

BOOST YOUR CHANCES:
LIFESTYLE CHANGES

Women and men who want to conceive can improve their chances by improving their lifestyles. Unhealthy lifestyle choices include smoking, drinking alcohol to excess and using illegal drugs – these behaviours have been shown to reduce fertility, negatively affect foetal health, and increase the risk of miscarriage. Though lifestyle changes may be hard, it is worth it for your own health as much as your baby's.

SMOKING

- Women who smoke are 1.5 times more likely than non-smokers to take more than a year to conceive

- The 7,000 chemicals in cigarette smoke (including nicotine) damage a woman's eggs and reproductive organs, creating problems with ovulation

- Smoking while pregnant increases the risk of premature birth, low birth weight and infant cot death

- Male smokers often have problems with erectile dysfunction, and their sperm is known to be damaged by smoking

ALCOHOL

- Studies have shown that women who consume more than six units of alcohol per week are 18 per cent less likely to conceive

- Even when a woman does conceive, excessive alcohol consumption can lead to foetal alcohol syndrome, an umbrella term for a range of abnormalities such as impaired growth, intelligence and sensory perception

- There is no known safe amount or safe time to drink alcohol during pregnancy

ILLEGAL DRUGS

- For some illegal drugs, the evidence on their harmfulness to fertility and pregnancy is clear; for others, less so

- Some studies indicate that cannabis use hinders ovulation in women (and smoking it is obviously harmful)

- The use of amphetamines, methamphetamine, cocaine and heroin has been linked to placental abruption (separation from the uterus) and miscarriage

BOOST YOUR CHANCES:
AVOIDING HAZARDS

The following factors, over time, may cause infertility or miscarriage by damaging egg cells or impairing your overall health. They should be avoided wherever possible.

However, rather than worrying too much, it is best to remember that the chances of any problems arising are small.

1 **X-rays**

at airports or during medical treatment

2

Long-haul flights

There is a higher likelihood of deep-vein thrombosis when you are pregnant (see pages 132–3 for travel tips)

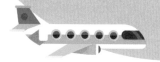

6 Bacteria in soil

Wear protective gloves if you're working in the garden

7 Chemical-based cleaning products

such as oven cleaner – wear protective gloves and take extra care not to inhale fumes

5 Cats and kittens

particularly their litter trays, as they can carry the bacteria that causes toxoplasmosis – a serious parasitic disease. Wear protective gloves

Livestock 4

especially pregnant sheep, can carry dangerous bacteria that may harm a developing foetus

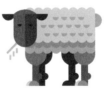

3 Chicken pox

especially if you haven't had chicken pox before, as this illness can cause complications for both mother and baby

If you have any concerns that you may have been exposed to any of the above risks, contact your doctor or midwife.

BOOST YOUR CHANCES: DIET

You are what you eat. If you want to have a healthy body that is ready to nurture a new life, then it is vital to pay close attention to what you eat and drink. Maintaining a healthy weight through diet and exercise will not only improve your chances of getting pregnant, but will also give your baby the best start in life. The same is true for men – a healthy lifestyle and diet improves sperm health. Both men and women should try to make any lifestyle and dietary changes at least two months before trying to conceive. For information on healthy eating after conception, see Chapter 3.

A BALANCED DIET FOR OPTIMUM FERTILITY

Fruit and vegetables

- Eat at least five portions a day, whether fresh, frozen, canned, juiced or dried
- An important source of vitamins and minerals – green, leafy vegetables are a particularly good source of folic acid

Protein

- Lean meat, fish, poultry, eggs, pulses, nuts, beans
- Eat two portions of fish a week, one of which should be oily fish

CALORIES – RECOMMENDED DAILY INTAKE

**WOMEN
2,000**

**MEN
2,500**

Men need more daily calories, not just because of their generally bigger size, but because of their greater muscle mass.

Starchy foods

- Potatoes, sweet potatoes, oats, wholemeal bread, rice, pasta, noodles
- Carbohydrates are important for energy, vitamins and fibre

Dairy

- Milk, low-fat yogurt, fromage frais, cheese
- An important source of calcium

Foods to limit

- Anything high in fat and/or sugar
- Crisps, chocolate, ice cream, pastries, cake, fizzy drinks

BOOST YOUR CHANCES: FOLIC ACID

If you are trying to conceive, a crucial element of your diet is your intake of folic acid. This should be taken as a vitamin supplement from the time you stop using contraception. Otherwise known as Vitamin B9, folic acid is also found in fortified foods such as breakfast cereals. You should also try to eat foods that are naturally rich in folic acid.

Why do I need folic acid?

Folic acid is necessary to prevent neural tube defects (NTD) in a developing embryo. The neural tube is the part of the embryo that will become the spinal cord and brain. Taking folic acid will help ensure the embryo develops correctly during the first 12 weeks after conception.

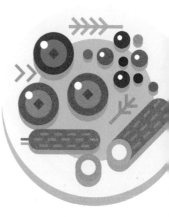

Dosage:

- Take folic acid at least two months before you start trying to conceive
- Take for at least 12 weeks into pregnancy
- Dosage: 0.4 mg every day

A higher dose of 5 mg is recommended if:

- You are taking other medication, e.g. for epilepsy, which may inhibit absorption of folic acid
- You have already had a child with a neural tube defect
- You have a BMI of over 30 (see page 36)
- You have a history of diabetes

Which foods contain naturally occurring folic acid?

- **Green, leafy vegetables**
- **Avocado**
- **Raspberries**
- **Citrus fruits**
- **Asparagus**
- **Beans, peas and lentils**
- **Brown rice**

Research has shown that increased intake of folic acid can prevent up to 70 per cent of cases of spina bifida.

BOOST YOUR CHANCES:
CALCIUM AND FATTY ACIDS

As well as increasing your intake of folate-rich foods and folic acid supplements, and eating a diet rich in vegetables and protein, you can enhance your chance of conceiving by eating plenty of foods high in fatty acids and calcium.

FATTY ACIDS

Fatty acids, otherwise known as the 'good' fats – Omega-3, Omega-6 and Omega-9 – are an essential part of a healthy diet, particularly when you are trying to conceive. The most important of these three fatty acids is Omega-3 in terms of fertility health.

Omega-3
- Regulates hormones, increases cervical mucus, and increases blood flow to the uterus
- Found in oily fish, such as mackerel, and in green, leafy vegetables

Omega-6
- Strengthens cell structure and reduces inflammation in the body
- Found in seeds, nuts and most vegetable cooking oils

Omega-9
- Helps strengthen the immune system and balance cholesterol levels
- Found in seeds, nuts and avocados, with highest levels in olive oil

CALCIUM

Recent studies have shown that calcium is vital for triggering the growth of the embryo. This mineral helps alkalise the cervix, creating a less hostile environment for both the sperm and the egg.
You should consume around 1,000 mg a day through eating dairy products and leafy greens, or with supplements

FERTILITY FOODS FOR MEN

Men also need to make sure their diet is full of fertility-boosting foods to ensure their sperm can tackle the long and difficult journey to fertilise the egg.

Zinc
- Keeps testosterone levels high and improves sperm health
- Found in red meat, pumpkin seeds, and vegetables such as peas

Folic Acid
- Studies have shown men with higher levels of folic acid have fewer abnormal sperm
- Highest levels found in asparagus and lentils

CoQ10
- An antioxidant enzyme found in nuts and seeds, particularly sesame seeds
- Taking a CoQ10 supplement can boost fertility by 13 per cent, as it helps the motility of the sperm

Selenium
- This antioxidant helps form healthy sperm and increases sperm motility
- Found in brazil nuts and fish such as salmon and tuna

Vitamin E
- Sperm quality is improved by having plenty of Vitamin E in your diet
- It is commonly found in almonds and other nuts

Vitamin C
- As well as helping with general health, Vitamin C increases both sperm count and the health of the sperm
- The best source is citrus fruits

Fatty Acids
- Omega-3 fatty acids are needed to produce plenty of prostaglandins in the semen. These suppress the female immune system's attack on the sperm when they enter the cervix
- Found in walnuts and oily fish such as sardines and salmon

CHAPTER 2

BEING PREGNANT

INTRODUCTION

You're officially pregnant! The implantation of the fertilised egg into the wall of your uterus sets off a chain reaction of events that will transform your body in many ways, both visible and invisible. For example, a surge in pregnancy hormones will safeguard the embryo inside you, making sure it has the best chance of developing into a healthy baby. It can be a very exciting time, both for you and the people around you. But you may also be curious or unsure about what's going to change. This chapter looks at a number of topics, debunking some of the myths about pregnancy as well as giving you some key facts about the changes ahead.

FROM EGG TO EMBRYO

Your baby-to-be will grow from a single cell into an embryo very quickly after fertilisation. Here's what it will look like as it develops and travels along your fallopian tube before attaching itself to the lining of your womb.

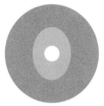 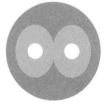 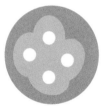

Fertilised egg →
0 hours after fertilisation

2-cell stage —
30 hours after fertilisation

4-cell stage —
45 hours after fertilisation

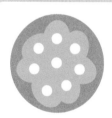 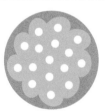 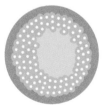

→ **8-cell stage** —
72 hours after fertilisation

→ **16-cell stage** —
96 hours after fertilisation

→ **Blastocyst stage (100+ cells)**
5 days after fertilisation

The fertilised egg is just about visible to the naked eye – roughly the size of a grain of sand (1 mm / 0.04 inches). Once it has reached the blastocyst stage, the process of differentiation will begin. This involves the cells dividing into three separate layers: the mesoderm, the ectoderm and the endoderm – with each layer being responsible for growing specific parts of your baby's body.

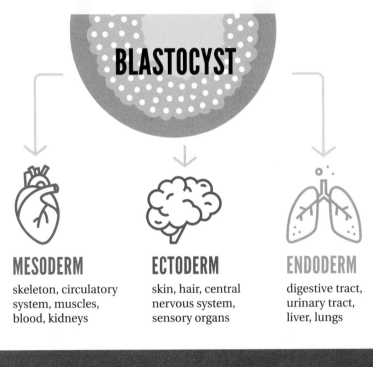

MESODERM
skeleton, circulatory system, muscles, blood, kidneys

ECTODERM
skin, hair, central nervous system, sensory organs

ENDODERM
digestive tract, urinary tract, liver, lungs

Once the blastocyst attaches itself to the uterus lining – in a process called implantation – the inner cells start to become the embryo and the outer cells start to become the placenta.

PREGNANCY MYTHS

MYTH | **You should eat for two**

- Non-pregnant women normally require around 2,000 calories a day

- When you're pregnant, this should increase by only 200–300 calories

- This is the equivalent of about two slices of brown toast spread with peanut butter

- After your baby is born, you may need up to 500 extra calories to help with milk production

- See Chapter 3 for more information on eating healthily while pregnant

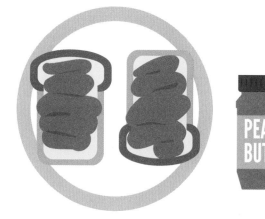

MYTH — Body lotion can help prevent stretch marks if applied regularly

- Stretch marks are caused when collagen fibres in your skin rupture because they cannot keep up with the rapid expansion

- Using body lotion will do little to prevent stretch marks, but it may help you to avoid the itchy, irritated feeling that accompanies them

- Cocoa butter or baby oil may be worth trying

MYTH — Your labour will start when your waters break

- Waters breaking means the rupture of the amniotic sac – the membrane around your baby – and the release of fluid

- Popular culture often depicts a woman who only realises she is going into labour when her waters break unexpectedly and dramatically, but this happens to just 1 in 10 women

- Most labours start with a gradual build-up of contractions, and in a number of cases the waters are broken by a medical professional once labour is well established

- In some cases, your waters can break much earlier than labour, with a wait of between 12 and 24 hours before labour becomes established – if contractions haven't started after 24 hours you may be induced

- Eating most fish in moderation is harmless during pregnancy as long as it has been frozen first (which kills parasites)

- Don't eat raw shellfish as it can cause food poisoning (some sushi contains raw shellfish)

- Cooked shellfish is safer, but you may decide to avoid it completely, as cooking is not guaranteed to remove all toxins

- It is important to avoid completely fish with high levels of mercury, such as swordfish, shark and marlin

- Tuna contains high levels of mercury: don't eat more than two tuna steaks a week (170 g / 6 oz raw or 140 g / 4.9 oz cooked) or four medium-sized cans a week (140 g / 4.9 oz when drained)

- Limit your intake of oily fish, such as fresh tuna, salmon, mackerel, herring, sardines, pilchards and trout, to two portions a week – this is due to the pollutants they may contain, despite the clear health benefits of eating oily fish

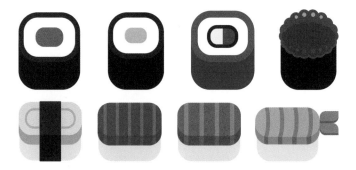

Morning sickness means you're having a girl

- There is no statistical correlation between fairly mild morning sickness and the gender of the baby

- However, recent studies (University of Washington, 2008) have suggested that in cases of extreme morning sickness, a female baby may be more likely

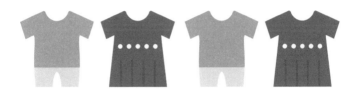

MYTH **You shouldn't dye your hair when pregnant**

- There is no reason to stop dyeing your hair during pregnancy

- Some women prefer to wait until the second trimester when the foetus is less vulnerable to harmful chemicals

- You could try using semi-permanent dyes, such as henna or vegetable-based dyes as these are largely chemical-free

MORNING SICKNESS

Morning sickness, sometimes known as NVP (nausea and vomiting during pregnancy), is one of the most common symptoms of pregnancy, although it is somewhat misnamed, since a woman can suffer from it throughout the day.

WHEN DO WOMEN GET MORNING SICKNESS?

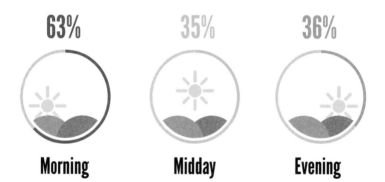

63%   **35%**   **36%**

Morning   **Midday**   **Evening**

HOW DOES MORNING SICKNESS AFFECT WOMEN?

43%

Affected their willingness to become pregnant again

48%

Affected their ability to take care of themselves

68%

Affected their general enjoyment of pregnancy

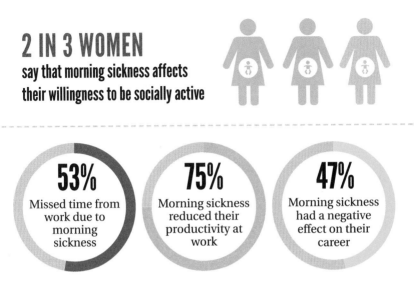

2 IN 3 WOMEN
say that morning sickness affects their willingness to be socially active

53%
Missed time from work due to morning sickness

75%
Morning sickness reduced their productivity at work

47%
Morning sickness had a negative effect on their career

Morning sickness can vary from simply feeling nauseous on waking up in the morning to full-blown hyperemesis gravidarum – where the mother-to-be must be hospitalised because she is unable to keep any food or liquid down. Morning sickness may have several possible causes, including hormonal changes, fluctuations in blood-sugar levels and the psychological impact of being pregnant.

- 9 out of 10 women will experience morning sickness in some form

- Around half of women experience vomiting as well as nausea

- Morning sickness usually improves between 14 and 16 weeks

- Around 5 per cent of women will experience morning sickness throughout their pregnancy

- 1 in 300 pregnancies cause hyperemesis gravidarum

MORNING SICKNESS: PREVENTION AND REMEDIES

There are several things you can do to both help prevent and alleviate morning sickness:

 Get plenty of rest, as tiredness can trigger nausea

 Try wearing acupressure bands on the wrists

3 Have some plain biscuits by your bed to eat as soon as you wake in the morning

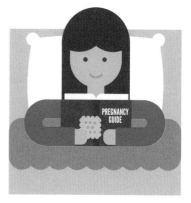

4 Avoid strong-smelling foods and chemicals

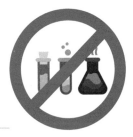

 5 Eat up to five small meals a day in order to keep the stomach full – hunger quickly turns to nausea

 6 Herbal teas, such as fennel, peppermint or camomile, may help

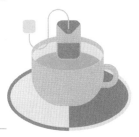

 7 Consuming anything containing ginger, such as tea, biscuits or flat ginger ale can help settle the stomach

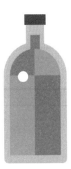

 8 Stay well hydrated – always keep a bottle of water with you

BABY DEVELOPMENT:
4 WEEKS

How Big?

Size of an apple seed
5 mm / 0.2 inches

How Heavy?

0.3 g / 0.01 oz

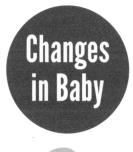

Changes in Baby

- The brain, spine and central nervous system begin to develop

- The amniotic sac is forming around the egg

- The baby's digestive tract is developing

Changes in Mother

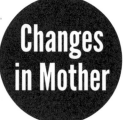

- Your total weight gain so far: 0.5 kg / 1 lb

- A surge of pregnancy hormones are produced to support the embryo

- As the fertilised egg implants, you may experience some mild bleeding

- You may be experiencing morning sickness and other early pregnancy symptoms

EARLY SIGNS OF PREGNANCY

Morning sickness is not the only sign that you are pregnant; there are multiple signifiers that appear in the first weeks of pregnancy that can indicate that your body has begun to grow a baby.

1 MISSED PERIOD

- One of the surest signs of pregnancy
- Your period may simply be late
- Most home pregnancy tests can provide a reliable answer

2 FATIGUE

- Pregnancy hormones may cause you to feel tired, upset or emotionally exhausted
- A common symptom but not a guarantee of pregnancy
- Tiredness may improve in your second trimester but return in the third

3 TENDER BREASTS

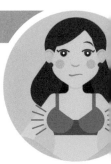

- Pregnancy hormones increase the blood supply to your breasts
- You may feel a tingling sensation around your nipples within a week of conception
- As this subsides, your breasts may become increasingly tender around six weeks, but this too will ease

4) FREQUENT URINATION

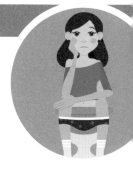

- You may feel the need to go to the toilet more often from around six weeks

- This is the result of pregnancy hormones, increased blood flow in your body, and your kidneys working harder

- Talk to your doctor if you feel pain or a burning sensation – this could be a urinary tract infection

5) METALLIC TASTE

- A metallic taste in the mouth is especially common in the first trimester

- This is due to the increase in your oestrogen levels

6) CRAMPS

- These may feel similar to pre-menstrual pains

- You may experience some spotting (pink or brown-coloured stains in your underwear) around the time you would have your period

- Believed to be the result of hormones and/or the egg implanting in your uterus

7) SMELL AND TASTE

- You may find you have an increased sensitivity to food smells

- A sudden dislike of strong flavours, such as coffee, spicy food and alcohol is also common

- Food cravings (see Chapter 3) may develop throughout pregnancy

CHANGES TO YOUR BODY:
PHYSICAL CHANGES

- Your breasts will grow in size to prepare for milk production

- Your organs (in particular, the intestines and lungs) will slowly be pushed up and back to accommodate the expanding uterus – this often results in breathlessness and indigestion

- The womb will expand from the size of a tennis ball (around 7 cm / 3 inches in diameter) to that of a watermelon at full term (around 60 cm / 24 inches in diameter)

- Your body will grow a whole new organ: the placenta (see pages 98–9)

- To support this new organ, the volume of blood being pumped around your body will increase by 50 per cent – and your blood vessels will expand to accommodate it

- The increase in blood flow often leads to a 'glowing' complexion

CHANGES TO YOUR BODY:
HORMONES

The changes experienced by a woman during pregnancy are largely caused by the ovaries' production of two key hormones: oestrogen (estrogen in American English) and progesterone.

The hormone hCG (human chorionic gonadotrophin) is released from the implanted egg and triggers the production of each pregnancy hormone.

Oestrogen levels shoot up during the first weeks of pregnancy. This doubles the blood supply to the uterus, thus producing a secure environment for the embryo. Oestrogen, along with progesterone, also swells the breasts as they prepare for milk production.

Progesterone has four main effects on the body during pregnancy:

- its sedative effect accounts for the extreme fatigue of the first trimester

- it relaxes your muscles and ligaments to help accommodate the expanding uterus

- it slows down your digestive system in order for more nutrients to be absorbed for the baby

- it thickens the cervical mucus – essential for keeping the baby safely in place

BABY DEVELOPMENT:
8 WEEKS

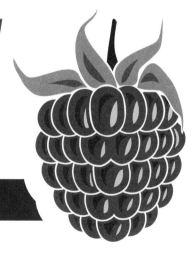

How Big?

Size of a raspberry
2.5 cm / 1 inch

How Heavy?

2 g / 0.07 oz

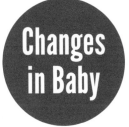

Changes in Baby

- The embryo can now be called a foetus

- Eyes, ears, nose and mouth are all forming into a recognisable face

- All major organs have now begun to develop

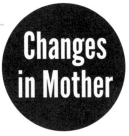

Changes in Mother

- Your total weight gain so far: 0.9 kg / 2 lb

- You may experience heartburn

- Food cravings are common at this stage

- You may be bloated due to a slowing down of the digestive system

CHANGES TO YOUR BODY: SKIN

Aside from stretch marks, created by the rapid expansion of the abdomen, it is quite normal for your skin to become more pigmented, due to your body's increased production of melanin. The darker your skin tone, the more prone you are to these changes, which include:

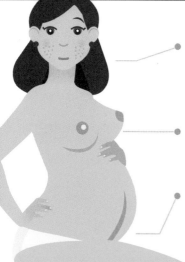

- patches of pigmentation on the face (known as melasma or the 'mask of pregnancy')

- a darkening of the skin around your nipples (areolae) and genitals

- the development of the dark brownish linea nigra (Latin for 'black line') from navel to groin

These skin changes are normal and not harmful, and they usually fade away after your baby is born, but always speak to your doctor or midwife if you have any concerns about changes to your body.

EMOTIONAL CHANGES

Heightened emotions are an inevitable part of pregnancy. The hormonal changes in the first trimester are the most dramatic your body has experienced since puberty, and the resultant mood swings are similar to a teenager's for a reason! These hormonal changes might manifest themselves in the following ways:

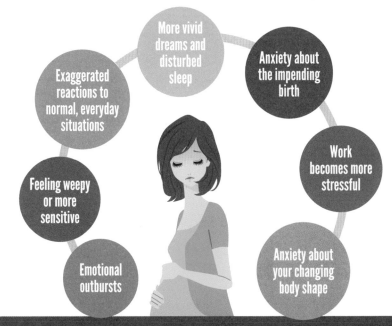

- More vivid dreams and disturbed sleep
- Anxiety about the impending birth
- Exaggerated reactions to normal, everyday situations
- Work becomes more stressful
- Feeling weepy or more sensitive
- Emotional outbursts
- Anxiety about your changing body shape

The best way to deal with these feelings is to acknowledge them and to talk to your partner, friends or family members who have been through the same thing. Always speak to your doctor if emotional changes are affecting your physical or mental well-being.

SHARING YOUR NEWS

The majority of couples choose to wait until the end of the first trimester (12 weeks) before telling everyone their news. Given that most miscarriages occur in the first 12 weeks, it seems sensible to wait. However, it may be hard to hide your pregnancy if symptoms such as morning sickness or fatigue are particularly extreme, and you may want to tell a few close friends, family or colleagues so that they can help out while being discreet. You may wish to tell people face to face, but increasing numbers of women are spreading the news via social media. Some fun ideas include:

- A photograph of a calendar with a picture of a baby on the due date

- A photograph of your baby scan superimposed over your bump

- Posting a picture of you and your partner's shoes, plus a pair of baby shoes, along with the caption 'Our family is growing by two feet'

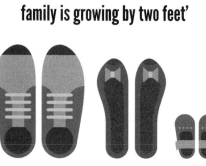

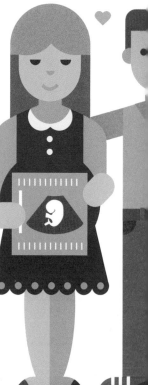

WHAT TO WEAR?

At first, you can accommodate your bump by wearing your baggier clothes, but as you grow, your current wardrobe will need some help.

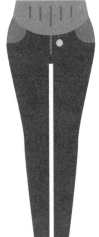

- Invest in a good pair of maternity jeans with a flexible front or side panel to accommodate your growing bump

- For more formal occasions or work, a wrap dress is a good investment as it can be let out as you grow

- A bump band or maternity bandeau will enable you to wear your own clothes for longer as it lets you undo the fastenings while keeping the garment in place

- Try borrowing maternity clothes or buying second-hand – they are worn for such a relatively short time, so they are often in good condition

- As your pregnancy advances, it is best to avoid high heels as they throw your posture out of balance – which makes the bump put even more pressure on your spine

- If you wear a uniform at work, ask for a larger size

- Your feet may expand as your ligaments relax, so you may need to buy some new shoes

- Your breasts will start to grow almost immediately and will continue to grow as the pregnancy progresses, so it's important to get a properly fitted bra

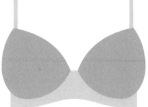

CHAPTER 3

NOURISHMENT

INTRODUCTION

Pregnancy is a big job for your body to take on – you are not only growing a human being inside you, but also a new organ, the placenta, to help nourish them. For this reason, it is vitally important to be at your optimum health and to properly nourish yourself when you're pregnant, for both your own benefit and your baby's. The food and drink you consume during pregnancy will have an effect, positive or negative, on your baby's health for the rest of its life. However, you shouldn't unduly worry if you slip up from time to time or treat yourself to the occasional indulgence. This chapter will give you some good advice and information on how eating well is one of the best things you can do while pregnant.

HEALTHY EATING TIPS

Here are six simple tips for eating well throughout pregnancy so that you achieve and maintain a healthy weight. If you keep this guidance in mind, you'll give yourself the energy and nutrients you need, and your baby will benefit in turn.

 Always eat breakfast – it's important fuel for the day ahead

 Watch portion size and frequency – eating smaller amounts throughout the day is better than binging before bed

 Base your meals on starchy foods – e.g. potatoes, bread, rice and pasta, and choose wholegrain varieties wherever possible

 Eat fibre-rich foods – this will improve your digestion and help you absorb important nutrients

 Eat your 5 a day – you should aim to consume at least five portions of fruit and vegetables a day (these can be fresh, frozen, canned, juiced or dried)

 Avoid or limit junk – cut out or at least cut down on fried foods and those that are high in sugar, salt and fat

HEALTHY WEIGHT GAIN

Although the commonly heard advice that you need to 'eat for two' is a myth, it's important to remember that too little weight gain during pregnancy is as bad as too much. If you are used to being very fit and lean, don't be afraid to let your body put on weight. You can always lose weight safely after birth through exercise and healthy eating. Also, if you don't gain much or any weight during the first three months of pregnancy because of morning sickness, don't worry. You will put on the most weight in the last half of your pregnancy.

Average normal weight gain during pregnancy

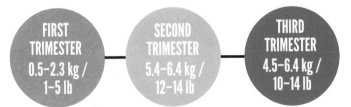

FIRST TRIMESTER
0.5–2.3 kg / 1–5 lb

SECOND TRIMESTER
5.4–6.4 kg / 12–14 lb

THIRD TRIMESTER
4.5–6.4 kg / 10–14 lb

Guidelines for total weight gain in pregnancy

Pre-pregnancy BMI	Classification	Recommended weight gain
< 18.5	Underweight	12.5–18 kg / 28–40 lb
18.5–25	Normal	11.5–16 kg / 25–35 lb
25–30	Overweight	7–11.5 kg / 15–25 lb
> 30	Obese	5–9 kg / 11–20 lb

BABY DEVELOPMENT:
12 WEEKS

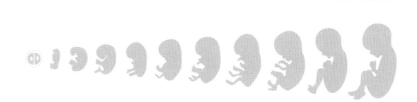

How Big?

Size of a lime
6.5 cm / 2.5 inches

How Heavy?

18 g / 0.6 oz

Changes in Baby

- Eyelids have developed and now cover the eyes

- Fingernails and toenails are now visible

- The sucking reflex has developed and the baby now swallows amniotic fluid

Changes in Mother

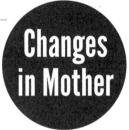

- Your total weight gain so far: 2 kg / 4.5 lb

- Morning sickness may start to fade

- You won't need to urinate as frequently

- Hormonal changes mean you may still feel quite emotional

NOURISHMENT FACTS

From conception to birth, over 40 weeks of development, a baby requires its mother to take in an extra:

- **925 g of protein –** equivalent to eating around three and a half whole chickens

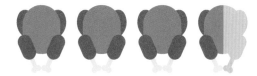

- **680 mg of iron –** equivalent to eating 34 kg / 75 lb of beef

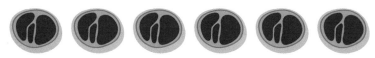

- **20–30 g calcium –** equivalent to drinking 25 litres / 5.5 gallons of milk

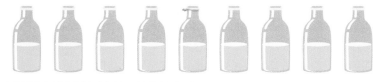

Slowed digestion during pregnancy means your body becomes more efficient at extracting nutrients from your food. For example, you will generally extract:

7%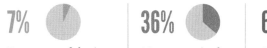

7 per cent of the iron in your diet in your first trimester

36%

36 per cent in the second trimester

66%

66 per cent in the third trimester

SUPERFOODS FOR PREGNANCY

Some foods are better than others at providing a good nutritional boost. Try to include the following superfoods in your diet regularly. If fresh produce is not available, frozen is just as good, as it preserves the nutrients. Note the vitamin and mineral content for each superfood.

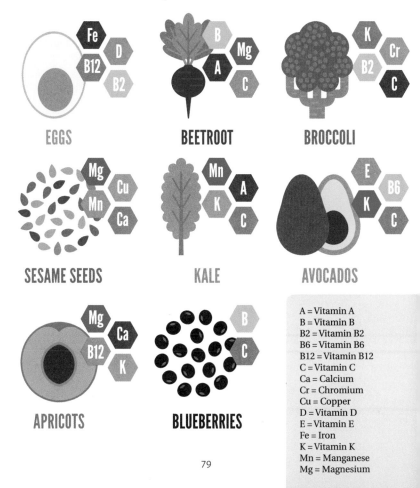

EGGS

BEETROOT

BROCCOLI

SESAME SEEDS

KALE

AVOCADOS

APRICOTS

BLUEBERRIES

A = Vitamin A
B = Vitamin B
B2 = Vitamin B2
B6 = Vitamin B6
B12 = Vitamin B12
C = Vitamin C
Ca = Calcium
Cr = Chromium
Cu = Copper
D = Vitamin D
E = Vitamin E
Fe = Iron
K = Vitamin K
Mn = Manganese
Mg = Magnesium

MACRONUTRIENTS: ESSENTIAL FOR ENERGY

PROTEIN — to serve as the building blocks of your body and baby

Requirement when pregnant: 51 g / 1.8 oz a day

Found in: lean meat, fish, chickpeas, tofu, beans

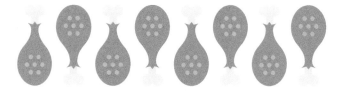

CARBOHYDRATES — for energy

Requirement when pregnant: roughly 50 per cent of your daily energy needs

Found in: wholemeal bread, pasta, rice

These are nutrients that you need to consume in relatively large quantities. They provide the essential energy for your body to function well and adapt to the needs of your growing baby.

FIBRE — to stabilise blood sugar levels and aid digestion

Requirement when pregnant: 18 g / 0.6 oz a day

Found in: bran flakes, dried fruit, wholemeal bread

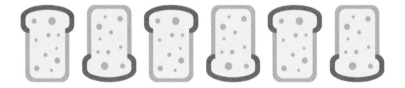

FATS (polyunsaturated) — to help absorb fat-soluble vitamins and energy

Requirement when pregnant: 30 g / 1 oz a day of Omega-3 and Omega-6

Found in: oily fish, flaxseeds, walnuts

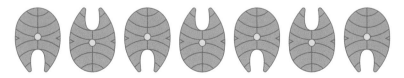

MICRONUTRIENTS:

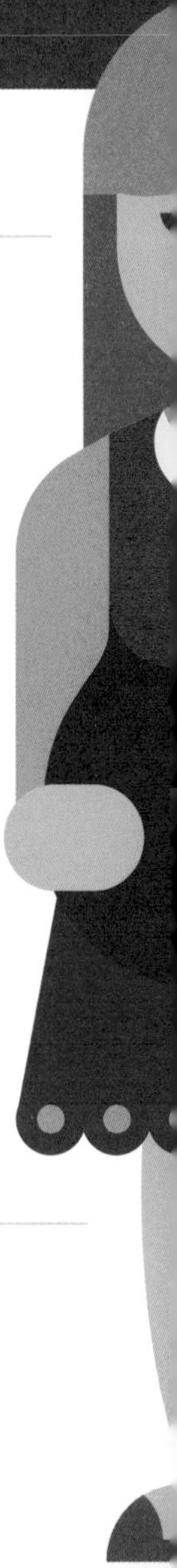

Vitamin A

0.7 mg per day

Needed for: immune system, eyes and baby's lungs

Sources: eggs, oily fish, milk, yogurt

Folic Acid

0.4 mg per day

Needed for: reducing risk of neural tube defects

Sources: best to take a folic acid supplement to guarantee correct intake

Vitamin B2

1.4 mg per day

Needed for: converting food into energy

Sources: milk, cheese, yogurt, spinach

Vitamin B6

1.2 mg per day

Needed for: metabolising protein

Sources: lean meat, fish

VITAMINS

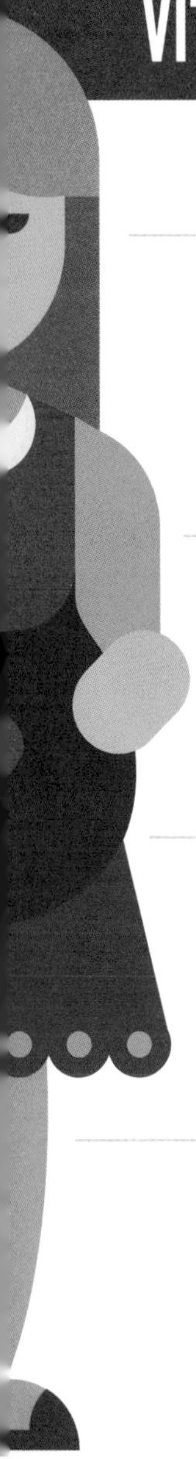

2.6 micrograms per day

Needed for: nervous system, processing folic acid, blood cells

Sources: all foods from an animal origin

Vitamin B12

85 mg per day

Needed for: cell health and absorbing iron

Sources: citrus fruits, potatoes, broccoli

Vitamin C

10 micrograms per day

Needed for: absorbing calcium

Sources: 15 minutes of sunlight or a dietary supplement

Vitamin D

3 mg per day

Needed for: repairing cell damage (but avoid high doses)

Sources: plant seed oils, nuts, eggs, fruit

Vitamin E

MUST-HAVE MINERALS

MINERAL	NEEDED FOR
Calcium	Bone building
Iron	Transportation of oxygen in the blood
Copper	Producing red and white blood cells
Magnesium	Metabolic functions
Zinc	Development of nervous and immune system
Selenium	Immune system and preventing cell damage
Potassium	Supports increase in blood volume
Manganese	Cell repair and making enzymes
Chromium	Balances glucose levels
Phosphorus	Strong bones and teeth, releasing energy from food

Along with vitamins, it is important to pay attention to the variety and volume of minerals that you are consuming during pregnancy. Though the amounts you need are small, they offer a wide range of essential benefits.

SOURCES	DAILY REQUIREMENT
Dairy products, sesame seeds, leafy green vegetables	800 mg
Meat, pulses, wholegrains, leafy green vegetables, dried fruit, nuts	14.8 mg
Nuts, peas, beans, beetroot	1.2 mg
Green leafy vegetables, nuts, seeds, fish, milk, peas, beans	270 mg
Red meat, pumpkin seeds	4–7 mg
Brazil nuts, walnuts, fish, meat, eggs	0.06 mg
Potatoes, beetroot, avocado, bananas	3,500 mg
Tea, nuts, cereals, lentils, raspberries	2.5 mg
Meat, wholegrains, lentils, broccoli, potatoes, spices	0.025 mg
Red meat, yogurt, milk, cheese, lentils, bread, oats	550 mg

HEALTHY SNACKING

It is always tempting to reach for something sweet when you are feeling hungry, never more so than during pregnancy when you seem to feel hungry all the time and yearn for an easy energy boost. However, it is much better to control your blood sugar levels and choose snacks that have high nutritional value and will keep you fuller for longer.

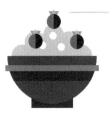
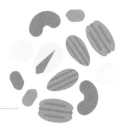

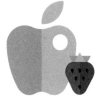
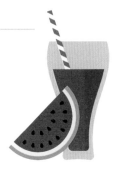

FRESH FRUIT

UNSALTED NUTS

**LOW-FAT YOGURT
WITH BLUEBERRIES**

DRIED APRICOTS

FRUIT SMOOTHIE
(NO ADDED SUGAR)

HUMMUS WITH
CARROT STICKS

UNHEALTHY FOOD

HEALTHY FOOD

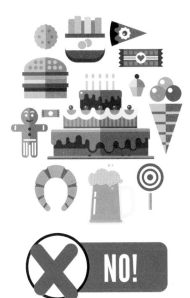

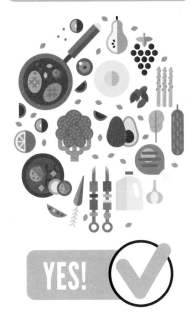

NO!

YES!

HEALTH ISSUES LINKED TO DIET

Several health issues may arise during pregnancy, ranging from the merely discomforting to the potentially dangerous. By carefully monitoring your diet and lifestyle, you can take steps towards preventing them altogether.

HEARTBURN

- Around 80 per cent of women will experience heartburn during pregnancy

- The oesophageal sphincter relaxes, letting stomach acid through

- Diet tip: avoid or limit large meals, fatty foods, citrus fruits and bananas

GESTATIONAL DIABETES

- Around 5 per cent of pregnant women develop gestational diabetes

- Hormones in the placenta affect the mother's production of insulin

- Usually develops around 24–28 weeks – your doctor will check your blood sugar levels

- If gestational diabetes causes you to have a particularly large baby, you are more likely to be induced early or have a caesarean section

- Diet tip: regulate blood sugar levels by eating low GI (glycaemic index) foods, which release energy slowly, and also avoid high-sugar foods altogether

CONSTIPATION

- Around 40 per cent of women will experience constipation in the first 14 weeks of pregnancy

- The body slows down digestion to increase the amount of nutrients it absorbs in the lower intestine

- Diet tip: drink plenty of water, eat fibre-rich foods, and try foods with a laxative effect, such as prunes and figs

PRE-ECLAMPSIA

- Around 3–5 per cent of women develop pre-eclampsia

- This is a serious condition relating to high blood pressure, usually during the second half of pregnancy

- More likely if you are overweight or over 35 years old

- More common in women who have low levels of antioxidants such as vitamins C and E

- Only around half of women know to look out for its symptoms, which include stomach pains, headaches, vomiting or feeling nauseous, seeing spots, swelling in your feet, ankles, face and hands, and gaining more than 2.3 kg / 5 lb in a week

- Diet tip: avoid or limit foods that exacerbate high blood pressure, such as caffeine and salt

FOOD SAFETY

Food safety has never been more important. Good food hygiene practices will help eliminate the risk of food poisoning, and careful food choices will ensure that you protect your baby from potential harm.

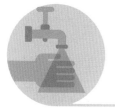

Wash hands thoroughly before any food preparation

Wash food thoroughly, especially if covered in soil, as it may contain harmful bacteria, which could cause toxoplasmosis

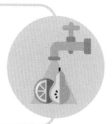

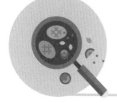

Serve cooked food at the right temperature – piping hot

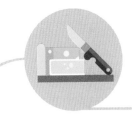

Avoid blue, soft and unpasteurised cheeses as they may contain harmful bacteria (e.g. listeria)

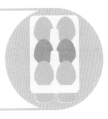

Never consume raw eggs or unpasteurised milk, due to the risk of salmonella and listeria

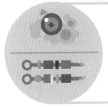

Always store meat products separately from foods to be eaten raw

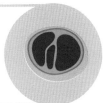

Never eat raw meat (including smoked, raw meats) as this may contain harmful bacteria

Store food at the correct temperature: below 5°C / 41°F for the fridge, and below -18°C / -0.4°F for the freezer

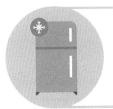

Avoid pâtés, as they may contain harmful bacteria

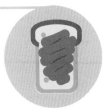

WHAT TO AVOID OR LIMIT

Some substances should be avoided or limited because they can have an immediate adverse effect on your baby when they pass from your bloodstream into your baby's body via the placenta.

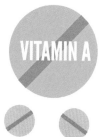

VITAMIN A

- Overconsumption of Vitamin A (more than 0.7 mg per day) can harm your unborn baby

- Avoid foods that contain high quantities, such as liver or liver products (e.g. pâté)

- Do not take dietary supplements that contain Vitamin A

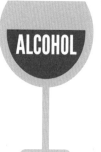

ALCOHOL

- Excessive consumption can lead to foetal alcohol syndrome, which affects around 1 per cent of births in the developed world

- Small amounts of alcohol may not cause any harm, but current advice is to avoid consumption of alcohol altogether

- Nearly half of women who routinely drink before pregnancy give up alcohol altogether, while nearly half cut down, and just 2 per cent make no change

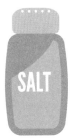

- Excessive consumption can lead to high blood pressure

- Try to consume no more than 6 g of salt per day

- Avoid or limit high-salt foods such as bacon, cheese, olives, pickles, soy sauce, yeast extract and gravy granules

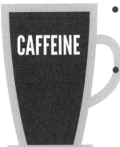

- You don't need to cut out caffeine completely, but it is recommended that you consume no more than 200 mg per day

- There is caffeine in not only coffee and tea, but other products such as chocolate and soft drinks

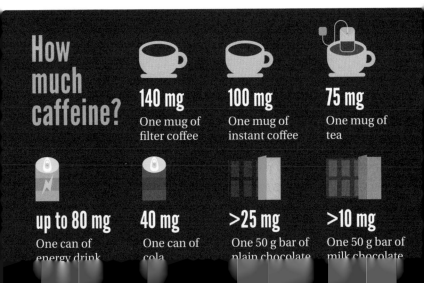

How much caffeine?

140 mg
One mug of filter coffee

100 mg
One mug of instant coffee

75 mg
One mug of tea

up to 80 mg
One can of energy drink

40 mg
One can of cola

>25 mg
One 50 g bar of plain chocolate

>10 mg
One 50 g bar of milk chocolate

BABY DEVELOPMENT:
16 WEEKS

How Big?

Size of an avocado
12 cm / 4.7 inches

How Heavy?

135 g / 4.7 oz

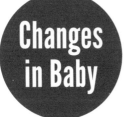

Changes in Baby

- Can now suck their thumb

- Hard bones are beginning to develop

- The neck is now distinguishable from the body

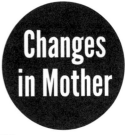

Changes in Mother

- Your total weight gain so far: 2.5 kg / 5.5 lb

- Changes in your skin pigmentation may appear

- Your bump will have grown enough for normal clothes to feel tight

COMMON CRAVINGS

When your body is craving certain foods, it is rarely for an arbitrary reason – more often than not it is a signal that your body is deficient in the vitamins or minerals that the craved food contains. Of course, if you are craving chocolate it may just be that your body is addicted to the sugar rush and comforting feelings that it provides, but other cravings are more complex.

Common Craving	What Your Body Wants	Healthy Suggestion
Chocolate	Magnesium Mg	Coconut
Sugary foods	Chromium Cr	Grapes
Starchy foods	Tryptophan (an amino acid)	Unsalted nuts
Oily foods	Calcium Ca	Organic milk
Salty foods	Sodium Na	Celery
Meat	Iron Fe	Pumpkin seeds

UNUSUAL CRAVINGS

Around 30 per cent of women experience cravings for non-food items, known as pica. The word 'pica' comes from the Latin for 'magpie' – a bird known for its ability to eat anything. If you find yourself craving any of the things below (apart from ice made from a clean water source), then it is crucial that you resist the urge: these substances contain toxins that are harmful to you and your baby. Speak to your doctor for advice on the nutrients that your diet may be lacking.

COMMONLY CRAVED PICA

- Soil or clay (geophagia)
- Ice (pagophagia)
- Purified starch (amylophagia)

OTHER PICA

- Pencil erasers
- Limescale
- Detergent
- Lead
- Coal
- Burnt matches
- Paper

POSSIBLE CONSEQUENCES

- Constipation
- Impacted colon
- Toxins passing through the placenta to your baby
- Parasitic infection (e.g. toxoplasmosis)
- Malnutrition (stomach struggles to absorb nutrient-rich food)

THE PLACENTA

Your baby gets all its nourishment from your bloodstream via the umbilical cord and the remarkable organ that is the placenta.

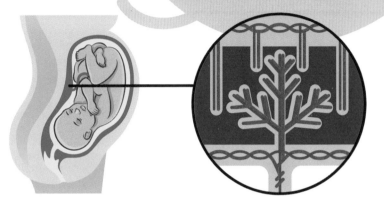

- The main umbilical vein (red) carries oxygenated blood as well as nutrients and the mother's antibodies to the foetus

- Two umbilical arteries carry away waste products such as carbon dioxide

- The three vessels coil around each other and are covered with a protective, jelly-like membrane

PLACENTA & UMBILICAL CORD FACTS

- Every minute, 20 per cent of your blood will flow through the placenta – equivalent to around 570 ml / 1 pint

- The capillaries in the placenta would reach 51 km / 32 miles if laid out in a straight line

- The umbilical cord will grow to 50 cm / 20 inches long

- By the third month of pregnancy, the placenta is fully developed

- It will weigh around 0.9 kg / 2 lb at birth

- The placenta contains around 1 litre / 0.2 gallons of amniotic fluid

- In the third trimester any antibodies you have are also passed on to your baby

- Amniotic fluid within the placenta provides a shock-absorbing, temperature-controlled environment. At 37.5°C / 99.5°F it is slightly warmer than your normal body temperature

- 1 in 80,000 babies are born 'in the caul' with the amniotic sac over their head – this was considered lucky in days gone by

- If unfurled, the surface area of the placenta would measure around 36 × 45 m / 120 × 150 feet

What happens to the placenta after birth?

- Some cultures, such as the Native American Navajo people, bury it

- A small number of people dry it out and convert it into pills to treat various ailments

- Some people choose to store blood from the umbilical cord in order to harvest stem cells in case of immunological illness

- Some cultures, such as the ancient Egyptians, viewed the placenta as sacred and built special tombs for royal placentas

- The stump of the cut cord will dry up and fall out of the navel 5–15 days after birth

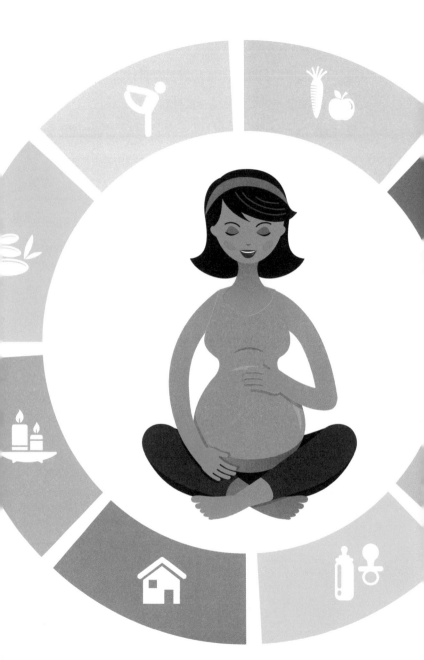

CHAPTER 4

WELL-BEING

INTRODUCTION

As well as eating a diet that nourishes you, now is the time to really try to take care of yourself in other ways – planning for the future, enjoying the present and avoiding undue stress.

The second trimester is the best time to really relish being pregnant – your morning sickness should have abated, along with the extreme fatigue of early pregnancy. Your bump is also a manageable size and most of the later discomforts of pregnancy, such as breathlessness and swollen ankles have yet to arrive.

EXERCISE
DURING PREGNANCY

There is no better time than pregnancy to establish a regular exercise regime. But if you are new to it, you must start gently and not overdo it. Exercise will not only help keep you in shape while pregnant, and make childbirth easier, but your baby will reap the benefits too, both now and in the future.

Try to do at least 30 minutes' moderate exercise 4 times a week.

Research indicates that you are 4.5 times more likely to need a caesarean section if you are not active during pregnancy.

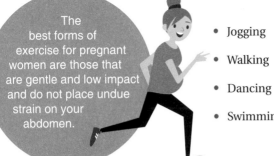

- Jogging
- Walking
- Dancing
- Swimming

- Pilates
- Yoga
- Cycling
- Moderate weight training

Exercise will increase the blood flow not only around your body, but also to the placenta.

The many discomforts that pregnancy brings can be alleviated by exercise.

Headaches

Cramps

Pelvic pain

Backache

Constipation

Stress and depression

Swollen feet

Ask your doctor or midwife before starting any new exercise regime – for some women, activities like yoga and Pilates can be too strenuous.

EXERCISE TO AVOID

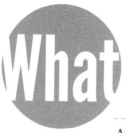

Activities involving rapid changes to your centre of gravity, such as squash or tennis

Anything that strains your pelvic muscles. For example, if using an exercise bike, ensure the resistance is not set too high

Anything that involves lying down for a long time

Scuba diving

Anything where you must lie on your stomach

Sit-ups

Contact sports, e.g. rugby

Anything that makes you dizzy

Any sport where there is a risk of falling, including horse riding and skiing

Any exercise that renders you unable to hold a conversation, e.g. running on a treadmill to the point where you are out of breath

DURING PREGNANCY

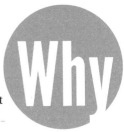
Why

→ As your posture and centre of gravity shift, it is harder to stay upright when weighted at the front

→ To avoid exacerbating pelvic pain (also known as symphysis pubis dysfunction or SPD)

→ To avoid disrupting the blood flow to the foetus by compression of the vena cava (the large vein into the heart)

→ Pressure underwater can affect the foetus. There is also an increased risk of decompression sickness when pregnant

→ To avoid damaging the foetus

→ Doing sit-ups incorrectly may contribute to a separation of the abdominal muscles, known as diastasis recti

→ To avoid abdominal trauma

→ Your blood flow can't keep up and you may faint

→ To avoid abdominal trauma

→ This is an indication that you are putting undue strain on your respiratory system

If you are weight training, you must be very careful to concentrate on the muscles that are not affected by an increase in relaxin – the hormone that loosens your ligaments in preparation for labour.

BABY DEVELOPMENT:
20 WEEKS

How Big?

Length of a banana
25 cm / 9.8 inches

How Heavy?

340 g / 12 oz

Changes in Baby

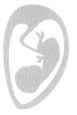

- Baby size is now measured from crown to heel rather than rump

- Hair is starting to grow on their head

- Teeth are developing inside their gums

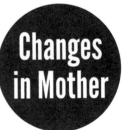

Changes in Mother

- Your total weight gain so far: 3 kg / 6.5 lb

- Your breasts may start producing early milk in the form of rich colostrum

- Joints and ligaments have relaxed so you may begin to feel more aches and pains

YOGA DURING PREGNANCY

Yoga and Pilates are both excellent ways of keeping fit and active while pregnant. The poses in these disciplines help you by stretching and strengthening your body, and the breathing exercises help you de-stress and relax.

Avoid the following if you are pregnant:

⊘ Deep forward bends with your legs closed

⊘ Deep twists

⊘ Extreme back bends and inversions

⊘ Yoga in a hot room (Bikram yoga) – the high temperatures are not good for a developing foetus and it may also cause you to feel light-headed and faint

Always talk to your doctor before beginning any new form of exercise. Everyone is different, and some women may have complications or historical health issues which could be exacerbated by doing yoga or Pilates. And if you start to feel dizzy, tired or unwell at any point, stop and rest.

The following positions are perfect in pregnancy – they will strengthen your muscles, improve posture and prevent back pain.

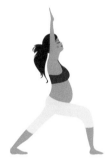

Warrior 1, 2 & 3:

To open up the chest and to lengthen and strengthen leg muscles

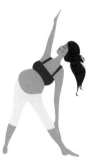

Triangle:

Great for relieving back ache and for strengthening your legs

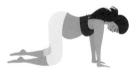

Cat/cow:

The best exercise you can do when pregnant – it eases back pain, increases blood flow to the pelvis and aids flexibility

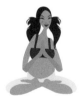

Bound angle:

Opens up the lower back and improves flexibility in the upper legs

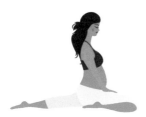

Pigeon:

This will release pressure from your sciatic nerve

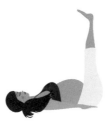

Legs up the wall:

An ideal way to relieve swollen ankles and help prevent varicose veins

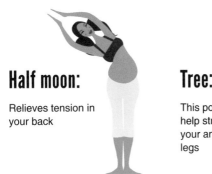

Half moon:

Relieves tension in your back

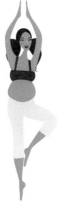

Tree:

This pose can help strengthen your ankles and legs

It is wise to attend a yoga class specifically designed for pregnancy to ensure you are able to practise these positions before you try them at home.

TESTS AND SCREENINGS:
FOR YOUR BABY

Depending on your healthcare provider, your baby's progress will be monitored at regular stages throughout the pregnancy. One of the key ante/prenatal appointments is based on an ultrasound scan – usually performed at around 12 weeks and 20 weeks. In the US, prenatal care is undertaken by an obstetrician while in the UK it is supervised by a midwife. Various countries have different schedules of care, but most will undertake the following tests and screenings.

Heartbeat

Using a Doppler machine, you will be able to listen to your baby's heartbeat while the medical practitioner checks for any abnormalities.

Around 3,000 babies are born every year with a congenital heart defect – and 1/3 of these are discovered during antenatal scans.

Amniocentesis

This test, which takes a sample of amniotic fluid by inserting a hollow needle into the uterus, can identify chromosomal disorders (e.g. Down's syndrome) and neural tube defects (e.g. spina bifida). It can also detect sickle-cell anaemia (an abnormality of the red blood cells). It is not a routine test for all pregnant women.

Quad Screen Blood Test

This picks up around 80 per cent of babies with either Down's syndrome or spina bifida. The test checks for the volume of four hormones in the blood:

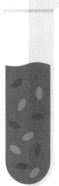

Alphafetoprotein (AFP)

Inhibin-A

Beta HCG
(human chorionic gonadotropin)

Oestriol

Ultrasound Scans

High-frequency sound waves are sent into your abdomen. When they hit solid bone or hard tissue it shows up as white, while soft tissue appears dark.

TESTS AND SCREENINGS:
FOR YOUR BABY

Various assessments can be made via ultrasound including:

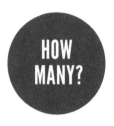

The scan will determine the number of foetuses that are developing inside the womb – whether it's a single baby, twins, triplets or more.

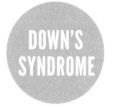

- This is a genetic defect where the baby has three copies of chromosome 21 instead of two.

- According to the World Health Organization, around 1 in every 1,000 babies born worldwide will have Down's syndrome. That's about 3,000–5,000 every year.

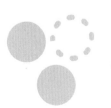

- A scan can detect extra fluid at the base of the baby's neck which suggests the possible presence of the trisomy gene.

- Around 50 per cent of babies with Down's syndrome will have features that can be picked up at a 20-week scan.

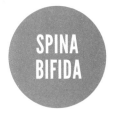

SPINA BIFIDA

- This is a genetic defect of the spine which can cause learning difficulties and paralysis of the baby's lower limbs.

- Around 95 per cent of babies with spina bifida will have features that can be picked up at a 20-week scan.

GENDER

At around 20 weeks it is possible to determine the gender of your baby from the ultrasound scan. Seventy-five per cent of prospective parents find out the gender at this stage.

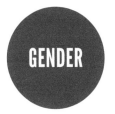

ESTIMATED DUE DATE

The crown–rump length (CRL) is the measurement from head to bottom that will help determine your baby's due date.

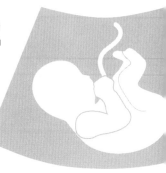

As a mother-to-be, you will also undergo a regular series of screenings to monitor your health. Your blood will be tested for the following:

Gestational Diabetes

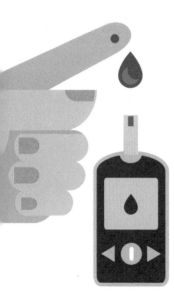

- This condition is a type of diabetes that affects women during pregnancy, resulting in blood sugar levels that are too high.

- It usually develops in the third trimester, is tested for at 24–28 weeks, and generally disappears after the baby is born.

- It affects around 5 per cent of women.

- If unchecked, it can lead to a larger baby and the greater likelihood of early induction or caesarean.

- Treatment options include diet, exercise and medication.

Blood Type

- You will find out your blood type, which is important if you need to have a transfusion for any reason following the birth.

- If you are rhesus negative (RhD negative), you may need extra care to lessen the risk of rhesus disease.

- Rhesus disease, also known as haemolytic disease of the foetus and newborn (HDFN), is a condition where antibodies in a pregnant woman's blood destroy her baby's blood cells.

- Most rhesus disease can be prevented by treatment during pregnancy or shortly after childbirth.

- Among Europeans, 16 per cent of the population are rhesus negative (though the prevalence among Basque people is about twice as high).

Anaemia

- This condition, which can cause you to feel tired, is the result of a deficiency of red blood cells or of the iron-rich protein haemoglobin in the blood.

- Tests will determine your red blood cell count. If it's too low, iron tablets will be prescribed.

- According to the World Health Organization's global data for 2011, 29 per cent of non-pregnant women and 38 per cent of pregnant women aged 15–49 years were anaemic.

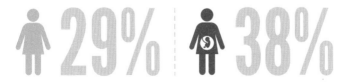

SLEEP **DURING PREGNANCY**

Sleep is incredibly important to good health, especially during pregnancy. Most pregnant women will experience disruption to their sleep, for a variety of reasons. Fortunately, there are plenty of simple methods that can help you get the rest you need.

Tips for Better Sleep

 Avoid caffeine and sugar

 Adjust bedroom temperature to be cooler than normal

 Avoid heavy meals and spicy food

 Try relaxation exercises, e.g. deep breathing and light stretching

 Avoid eating two hours before bedtime

 Buy a special elongated pregnancy pillow to go between your legs and support your bump

 Get enough fluids

 Take a warm bath or shower

 Develop a regular sleeping routine

Do not take any sleep aids. This includes over-the-counter medicines and herbal products.

They are not recommended for pregnant women. Always consult a doctor before taking any medicines during pregnancy.

BY THE END OF PREGNANCY, MORE THAN 9 OUT OF 10 WOMEN EXPERIENCE UNSETTLED SLEEP DURING THE NIGHT

Causes of Bad Sleep

- Fatigue
- Morning sickness
- Emotional turbulence
- Heartburn

- Restless leg syndrome
- Frequent urination
- Hip, shoulder and back pain

78% OF WOMEN EXPERIENCE MORE DISTURBED SLEEP DURING PREGNANCY THAN AT OTHER TIMES

SEX DURING PREGNANCY

Sex during pregnancy is healthy (except in the case of some health conditions, such as an incompetent cervix). An increase in hormones and the liberation from worrying about birth control means that you may feel keener on sex than ever before. However, it is worth bearing in mind that some positions should be avoided – particularly those that put any pressure on the bump.

MYTHS AND TRUTHS ABOUT SEX DURING PREGNANCY

MYTH **TRUTH**

Having sex will hurt the baby $\longrightarrow$ The uterus is sealed so sex is safe

The baby will be traumatised $\longrightarrow$ The baby has no idea what is happening

The baby could get infected $\longrightarrow$ The amniotic sac protects the baby from outside germs

Sex will induce labour $\longrightarrow$ Contractions from sex and orgasm will only bring on labour if your body is ready

BENEFITS OF SEX DURING PREGNANCY

- Burns calories
- Speeds up recovery after birth
- Improves sleep
- Reduces blood pressure
- Boosts immunity
- Increases intimacy

The following positions are ideal for a pregnant woman as they avoid any pressure on the abdomen and put the woman in control so that she feels comfortable:

Woman on top

Reverse cowgirl on a chair

Edge of the bed

Reverse cowgirl on a bed

Spooning

THE FINANCIAL COST **OF PREGNANCY**

Aside from medical costs, if you choose to go private or your insurance does not cover certain aspects of pregnancy, there are certain costs to take into account when pregnant.

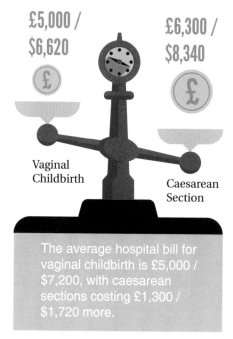

£5,000 / $6,620

£6,300 / $8,340

Vaginal Childbirth

Caesarean Section

The average cost of raising a child to the age of 21 is £222,000 or $294,000.

The average hospital bill for vaginal childbirth is £5,000 / $7,200, with caesarean sections costing £1,300 / $1,720 more.

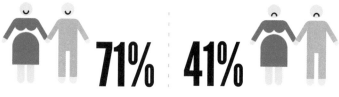

71% **41%**

71 per cent of couples say they feel financially prepared for parenthood, while 41 per cent of parents say that with hindsight they were not as prepared as they thought.

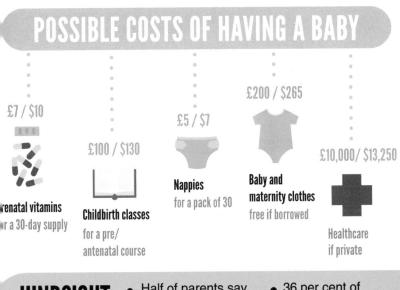

POSSIBLE COSTS OF HAVING A BABY

£7 / $10

Prenatal vitamins
for a 30-day supply

£100 / $130

Childbirth classes
for a pre/
antenatal course

£5 / $7

Nappies
for a pack of 30

£200 / $265

**Baby and
maternity clothes**
free if borrowed

£10,000/ $13,250

Healthcare
if private

HINDSIGHT

- Half of parents say they spent more money on car seats than necessary.

- 36 per cent of parents say they think they overspent on their buggy.

Essential items for newborns

Except for car seats – which you should buy new so that you are certain they are completely safe and undamaged – all of these items can be bought second-hand or borrowed. They are often barely used and will save you a lot of money.

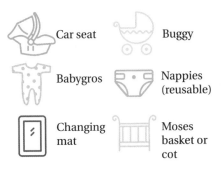

Car seat

Buggy

Babygros

Nappies
(reusable)

Changing
mat

Moses
basket or
cot

BABY DEVELOPMENT: 24 WEEKS

How Big?

Length of an ear of corn
33 cm / 13 inches

How Heavy?

570 g / 1.25 lb

Changes in Baby

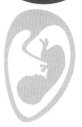

- Sweat glands are forming under the skin

- You will be able to feel your baby coughing and hiccupping

- They will start to really stretch and kick their legs and arms

Changes in Mother

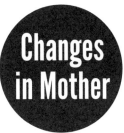

- Your total weight gain so far: 4.5 kg / 10 lb

- Your face and body may become puffy as you retain more water

- The area around your nipples (areola) will become more prominent

WORK AND CAREER

You have a responsibility to your employer to let them know that you are pregnant. Most women wait until after their 12-week scan to tell everyone, but you must inform your employer by the time you are around 6 months pregnant.

Tips for pregnancy at work

 Seek out a mentor or friend at work for support. Choose someone who has had a baby and will know the ropes

 Go through your job with your manager to assess any risks or health and safety issues

 You are entitled to take time off work for antenatal appointments

 Ask what maternity and paternity benefits your company provides

 Make sure there is enough time, before you leave your role, to train whoever will be your maternity cover

Experiences of pregnancy at work

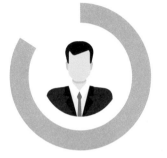 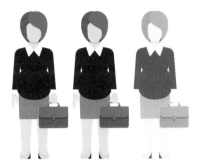

84% OF EMPLOYERS

believe that supporting pregnant workers and those on maternity leave is good for their business. The main benefit is their staff stay with the business longer.

2 OUT OF 3

women feel that they have enough support from their employer during pregnancy and when they return to work.

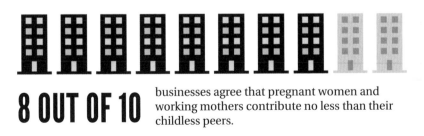

8 OUT OF 10

businesses agree that pregnant women and working mothers contribute no less than their childless peers.

DISCOMFORT IN LATE PREGNANCY

Pregnancy is a time of joy and excitement for what's to come, but it is also a time when the number of small discomforts and inconveniences can seem endless, especially towards the third trimester. Most of them will be due to your baby pushing against your bladder, diaphragm and other internal organs. Here are some common complaints…

 of women experience itchier skin when pregnant

 of pregnant women report numb fingers, due to carpal tunnel syndrome (compression of a nerve in the hand)

 of women suffer from varicose veins

 of women will suffer from stress incontinence

30% of women will suffer from a blocked nose

 25% of women will experience nosebleeds

 50%+ of women will get piles or haemorrhoids

 75% of women will feel breathless

 25% of women experience restless leg syndrome

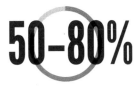 **50-80%** of women will suffer from swollen ankles or oedema (the build-up of watery fluid) in the third trimester

TRAVELLING
DURING PREGNANCY

You may want to make the most of your last months of freedom for a while by going on a trip with your girlfriends or your partner (known as a Babymoon). But you should choose the best time to go.

Travelling by car

When travelling by car, always wear your seat belt and make sure it's fitted correctly around your bump. If you're going on a long car journey, make sure you get plenty of breaks in order to stretch your legs.

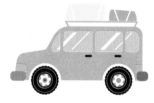

Travelling by train

Some train companies allow pregnant season-ticket holders to travel in First Class.

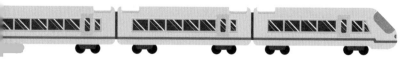

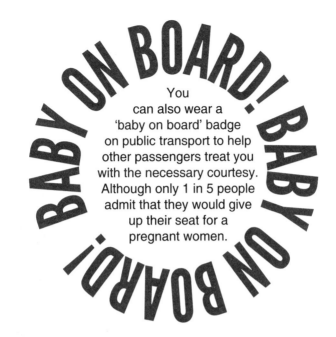

You can also wear a 'baby on board' badge on public transport to help other passengers treat you with the necessary courtesy. Although only 1 in 5 people admit that they would give up their seat for a pregnant women.

BABY ON BOARD! BABY ON BOARD! BABY ON BOARD!

How to fit your seat belt correctly

1 Strap the lap section of the belt across your thighs and under your bump, not across it (as the pressure across your belly could cause damage).

2 The diagonal shoulder section should go across your collarbone, between your breasts.

3 Fasten it so that it sits above your bump, not over it.

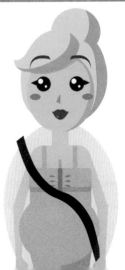

131

When to Travel

Weeks 1–12

- Inadvisable to travel long distances
- Higher risk of miscarriage
- Fatigue and sickness are at their worst

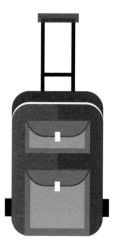

Weeks 13–28

- The best time to travel
- Risk of miscarriage is far smaller
- You have more energy

Weeks 29–40+

- Best to stay close to home, in case of premature labour
- Many airlines and ferry companies require a doctor's letter if you wish to travel after 28 weeks

Flying is inadvisable after 36 weeks due to the increased risk of deep vein thrombosis (DVT)

From 37 weeks, you have a higher chance of going into labour (34 weeks if you are carrying twins)

Travel Checklist

✓ Check whether you need vaccinations for your destination

✓ Double-check that your travel insurance policy covers you for any complications relating to pregnancy (most do but it's advisable to call up and check or read the small print in your policy)

✓ Avoid travelling to countries for which you need inoculations for malaria as they are incompatible with pregnancy

✓ If you are travelling somewhere hot, remember that you're more susceptible to sunburn during pregnancy – so make sure that you use a high factor suncream, cover up your skin and stay in the shade in the midday sun

✓ Check what medical facilities are close to your accommodation in case you need them

✓ If you're flying long distance, make sure you get up every 30 minutes for a quick walk up and down the cabin, to help prevent DVT

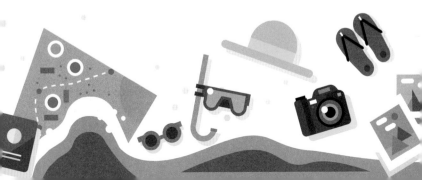

BABY DEVELOPMENT: 28 WEEKS

How Big?

Length of a cucumber
37 cm / 14.5 inches

How Heavy?

1 kg / 2.2 lb

Changes in Baby

- Hearing is well developed

- Eyes have become unsealed and can now sense light and dark

- Lungs are now mature enough to be able to work outside the womb (with a little help)

Changes in Mother

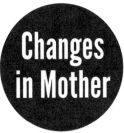

- Your total weight gain so far: 9 kg / 19 lb

- You may be experiencing heartburn, indigestion and cramps

- You may feel some faint but false contractions

- You may have red stretchmarks on your stomach

WAYS TO RELAX

The larger your bump, the more you will feel the need to give your body a break from the normal routine. There are many ways you can make yourself feel better, but now, more than ever, you deserve some relaxation.

MASSAGE

You don't have to stop having massages because you are pregnant, especially when they will improve your circulation and any muscle aches. Most beauty therapists now offer a mum-to-be massage. Therapists will either:

- Have you lie on your side with a pillow to support your head

- Or you can lean against an elevated massage table with pillows to support your upper back.

AVOID:

 Massage of the abdomen, as the pressure on the womb may harm your baby

 Acupressure points on the ankles, as these may stimulate contractions

Deep tissue massage, as this may dislodge a blood clot that could seriously harm your health

Wormwood, rue, oak moss, *Lavandula stoechas*, camphor, parsley seed, sage, clary sage and hyssop essential oils, as they may trigger contractions or cause bleeding in your womb

SWIMMING

Swimming is an excellent method of exercising and relaxing while pregnant, especially as the water takes the weight off your bump and can help ease your aches and pains. Check for antenatal classes at your local pool.

AVOID:

⊘ Exercising in pools where the water temperature is above 32°C / 89.6°F

⊘ Bathing in hydrotherapy pools (a special warm shallow pool) where the water temperature is above 35°C / 95°F

⊘ Spending time in steam rooms and hot tubs, as they may lead to overheating, dehydration and fainting – some hot tubs can be as warm as 40°C / 104°F

CHAPTER 5

FINAL STAGES

INTRODUCTION

You've reached the final straight – there are just a few weeks to go before your baby arrives. Now is the time to make final preparations, such as practising setting up your buggy and installing the car seat, packing a hospital bag, preparing a birth plan and working out the best route to the hospital. Indulge the urge to nest and get your home prepared for the new arrival. But the most important thing to do now is stay calm – try to avoid stress at all times, as it can hinder the release of oxytocin, which is a vital hormone for ensuring a smooth birthing experience.

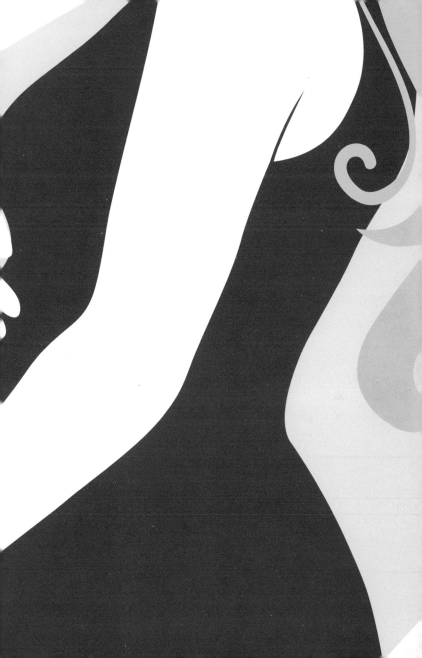

PREPARATIONS
IN THE LAST FEW WEEKS

In the weeks running up to your due date, take a bit of time to make your final preparations before the baby arrives. Many working women take up to a month off before their due date, depending on their job and their health.

PRACTISE:
- Relaxation (see pages 136–7)
- The route to hospital
- Putting the car seat in the car
- Setting up your buggy or pram

TO DO:
- ✔ Pack your hospital bag (see pages 144–5)
- ✔ Finalise your birth plan
- ✔ Attend antenatal classes
- ✔ Make lots of meals for your freezer
- ✔ Get your hair cut

If you can take time off work, do. Based on studies in the US and UK, research by the University of Essex in 2012 found that women who worked after they were eight months' pregnant had babies on average around 230 g / 0.5 lb lighter than those who stopped work between six and eight months.

PREPARING THE NURSERY

There is no need to have a complete nursery all ready for when you get home from hospital. Most babies start their lives by sleeping in their parents' room. But you may want to prepare a dedicated changing space.

A low light source for night feeds – so as not to startle or fully rouse the baby when they need a night feed or nappy change

A hip-height chest of drawers or changing station with handy storage for nappies, cotton wool, spare sleepsuits, etc.

A comfortable chair – for breastfeeding

A plastic changing mat with padded sides

A sleeping bag for the baby – although these are not recommended for newborns

An ideal temperature of 16–20°C / 61–68°F

Measures to reduce noise and draughts from outside

Blackout blinds – to help aid sleep

The Lullaby Trust, which promotes safer sleep for babies, recommends that babies should sleep in a Moses basket or a separate cot in the same room as you for the first six months. This significantly reduces the risk of sudden

BABY DEVELOPMENT: 32 WEEKS

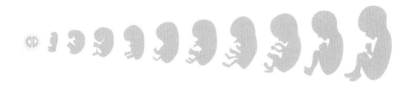

How Big?

Length of a pineapple
40.5 cm / 16 inches

How Heavy?

1.6 kg / 3.5 lb

Changes in Baby

- Really putting on weight, gaining a third of their body weight in the last seven weeks of pregnancy

- Should now start moving into position ready for birth – head down

Changes in Mother

- Your total weight gain so far: 11 kg / 24 lb

- Your bellybutton will be stretched out and flattened by now

- Your pelvic joints and the base of your ribcage may be sore

- You may feel breathless or need to urinate more due to the baby pressing on your internal organs

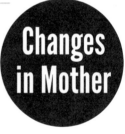

WHAT TO PACK IN YOUR HOSPITAL BAG

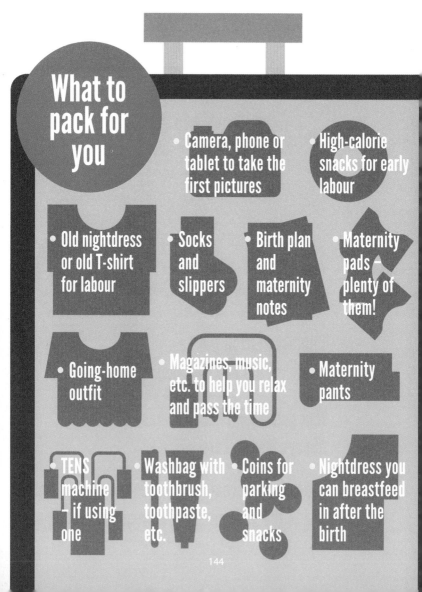

What to pack for you

- Camera, phone or tablet to take the first pictures
- High-calorie snacks for early labour
- Old nightdress or old T-shirt for labour
- Socks and slippers
- Birth plan and maternity notes
- Maternity pads – plenty of them!
- Going-home outfit
- Magazines, music, etc. to help you relax and pass the time
- Maternity pants
- TENS machine – if using one
- Washbag with toothbrush, toothpaste, etc.
- Coins for parking and snacks
- Nightdress you can breastfeed in after the birth

Have your hospital bag packed and ready at hand from at least 36 weeks, just in case you go into labour early.

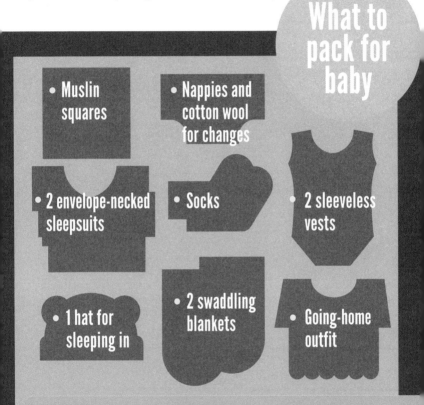

What to pack for baby

- Muslin squares
- Nappies and cotton wool for changes
- 2 envelope-necked sleepsuits
- Socks
- 2 sleeveless vests
- 1 hat for sleeping in
- 2 swaddling blankets
- Going-home outfit

Dads, you should pack some entertainment essentials too – you may have a long wait on your hands. Don't forget to pack a charger for your phone – you don't want to have the battery run out just before you try to take your first photo! Also, pack a bag with a change of clothes, some snacks and drinks, and swimwear (if you want to go into the birth pool for a water birth). Finally, don't forget the car seat.

SIGNS OF
APPROACHING LABOUR

1 A few weeks before labour, your bump will start to 'drop' into your pelvis. Also known as 'lightening', this process is how the baby gets into position to be born.

2 Your breasts will swell and may start leaking colostrum – the nutrient-rich early breast milk.

If you're getting wet patches on your clothes, buy some disposable breast pads that you can pop inside your bra.

3 You may experience Braxton Hicks contractions, which result from a hardening of the uterus. These infrequent and irregular contractions should last no longer than 30 seconds and occur no more than three or four times a day – any more than this and you should contact your midwife or doctor.

4 You have a show, which is when the mucus plug covering your cervix in pregnancy becomes loose and you notice a brown, pink or red-tinged stringy or jelly-like discharge. The plug can come out either in one piece or more gradually over several days.

Let your midwife know if you experience discharge. If the discharge is bright red, or heavy, go straight to hospital.

5 Diarrhoea – this is not a symptom that all women experience, but it can happen as you're nearing labour because the hormones that help your uterus contract can also cause a loosening of the bowels.

It's important to stay hydrated – especially if you're having regular toilet stops – but avoid diuretic drinks, such as caffeinated coffee and tea, and fruit drinks which can irritate the bladder.

6 Frequent urination – as the baby gets into position in the birth canal, the discomfort of it pressing against your bladder can seem worse than ever before.

WHEN TO GO INTO HOSPITAL

You should contact the labour ward if the following things have happened:

 1 Your waters have broken. But note that only about 15 per cent of women begin labour in this way

 2 Contractions are regularly 5 minutes apart and 1 minute in duration

HOW LONG DOES LABOUR LAST?

- Generally, but not always, labour tends to last longer for first-time mothers

- Labour may take around 12–14 hours for first-time mothers, but may last much longer

- Labour may take about 8 hours for women who have given birth before

- Remember: the exact duration varies greatly from one woman to another

BABY DEVELOPMENT: 36 WEEKS

How Big?

Length of a head of celery
46 cm / 18 inches

How Heavy?

2.5 kg / 5.5 lb

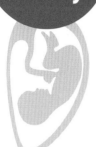

Changes in Baby

- The head will descend into the pelvis in preparation for birth

- Nails have now grown beyond the tips of their fingers

- If a boy, his testicles will have descended

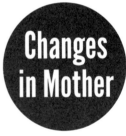

Changes in Mother

- Your total weight gain so far: 12 kg / 26 lb

- Your bump will appear lower down on your body

- Once the baby drops into the pelvis, heartburn and breathlessness may lessen

- Your bladder will feel under pressure and you will need to urinate more frequently

BEING OVERDUE

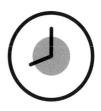

280 The average pregnancy lasts 280 days

Only 5 per cent of babies arrive on their estimated due date (EDD)

If nothing has happened 10–14 days after your EDD, induction is recommended

8 IN 10 BABIES
in the UK are born between 38 and 42 weeks of pregnancy

1 IN 100 WOMEN
will not have given birth within four weeks of their due date

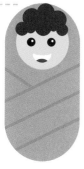

Babies born past their due date are usually:

Larger

More alert

Have more hair

Have lost their vernix (the waxy substance coating their skin)

In 1945, Beulah Hunter, a 25-year-old woman from Los Angeles, had a baby daughter whose gestation period was reported to have been 375 days.

Reasons for induction:

 If you are overdue

 If your waters have broken

 If you or your baby has a health problem

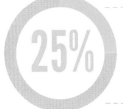 **Around 25 per cent of births are induced in developed countries**

Methods of medical induction

- Prostaglandin pessaries (on average, 2–3 will be needed)
- Artificial rupture of the membranes (known as a cervical sweep)
- Artificial oxytocin (Syntocinon) administered via a drip

Methods of non-medical induction (there is no real proof that these work)

- Reflexology, acupressure and aromatherapy
- Drinking castor oil or raspberry leaf tea, or eating a very spicy meal
- Sex – the prostaglandins contained in semen may help in the same way as medical pessaries

HOME BIRTHS

The place where women in the developed world have given birth has changed a great deal over the last century. At the beginning of the twentieth century, most babies were born in the family home, helped into the world by a midwife. By the 1950s, births were increasingly medicalised, with doctors taking over the birth. Today, although only a small percentage of births occur at home, there is an increasing movement towards midwife-led care, and many more women are giving birth at home.

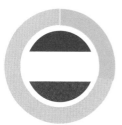

The Netherlands has the highest percentage of home births: 29%

You may need to transfer to a hospital if there are complications (such as bleeding) – the 2011 Birthplace study found that 45 out of 100 women having their first baby at home were transferred to hospital, compared with only 12 out of 100 women having their second or subsequent baby.

Home Births in the UK

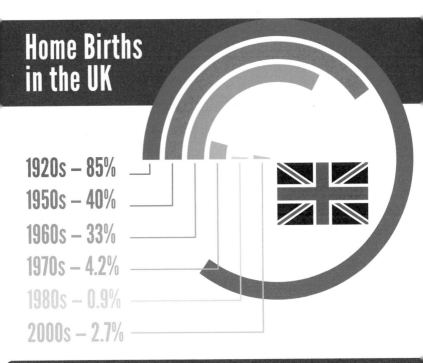

1920s – 85%
1950s – 40%
1960s – 33%
1970s – 4.2%
1980s – 0.9%
2000s – 2.7%

If you are considering having a home birth, always discuss the necessary preparations and possible risks with a trained doctor or midwife – this will help you make an informed decision on what is best for you and your baby.

For women having their first baby, home birth slightly increases the risk of a poor outcome for the baby (from 5 in 1,000 for a hospital birth to 9 in 1,000 – almost 1 per cent – for a home birth).

For women having their second or subsequent baby, a planned home birth is as safe as having your baby in hospital or a midwife-led unit.

HOSPITAL BIRTHS

Most women in the developed world today give birth in hospitals. For women with certain medical conditions, it is definitely safest to give birth in hospital because specialists are available if you need extra help during labour.

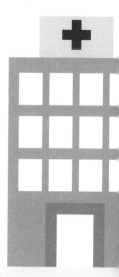

Place of birth in the UK (2013)

Total births 690,820

NHS establishments	At home	Non-NHS establishments	Elsewhere
97.2%	2.3%	0.3%	0.2%
671,638	15,552	2,248	1,382

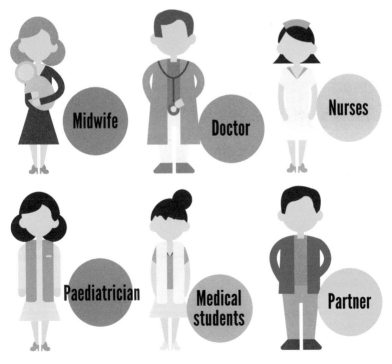

More than 8 in 10 fathers attend the birth of their baby

Who might be present at a hospital birth?

Midwife

Doctor

Nurses

Paediatrician

Medical students

Partner

BABY DEVELOPMENT:
40 WEEKS

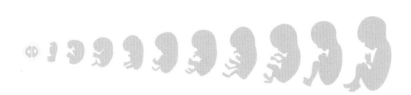

How Big?

Size of a watermelon
51 cm / 20 inches

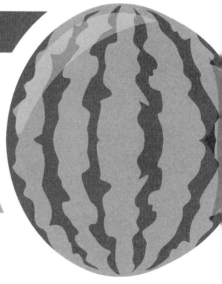

How Heavy?

3.4 kg / 7.5 lb

Changes in Baby

- The protective white fat on the baby's skin (vernix) will disappear

- The layer of fine hairs (lanugo) will have fallen out

- The baby's first bowel movement, known as meconium, will develop in the intestine

Changes in Mother

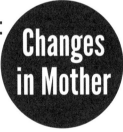

- Your total weight gain so far: 13 kg / 28 lb (weight tends to remain static in last few weeks of pregnancy)

- You may start to feel irregular Braxton Hicks contractions as your cervix prepares for birth

- Your nesting instinct may go into overdrive

CAESAREAN SECTIONS

The caesarean section was not named after Julius Caesar, but after the Roman law (Lex Caesarea) that decreed a child must be cut out and saved if the mother was dying or dead. It was intended as a last resort due to the almost 100 per cent mortality rate. Even by the nineteenth century, mortality for the mother was around 75 per cent. Today, in the developed world at least, the mortality risk is minuscule and the operation is very safe.

Types of C-section

Elective (planned) caesarean – **40%** **(mother is given an epidural)**

Emergency (unplanned) caesarean – **60%** **(mother is given general anaesthetic)**

Reasons for an elective C-section

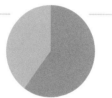

- Mother has previously had a caesarean and there were complications
- Baby is in a bottom-down (breech) position
- Baby is in a sideways (transverse) position
- Multiple births – twins, triplets or more
- A low-lying placenta (placenta praevia)
- Severe pre-eclampsia
- Heart problems
- Viral infections
- Mother's personal choice

Reasons for an emergency C-section

- Baby becomes distressed during labour

- Labour is too long and slow

- Attempts to use other instruments (e.g. forceps) have failed

- Placenta has come adrift (placental abruption)

- A previous caesarean scar ruptures (very rare)

- Umbilical cord is pushed out first (prolapse of the cord)

Typical C-section duration: 35–45 mins

 Delivery:
5–10 mins

 Repairing the uterus and abdomen:
30–40 mins

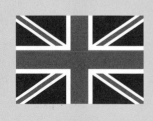 In the UK in the 1920s, 1 in 200 births was a caesarean – and these operations tended to be carried out only if the baby was too big for the mother's pelvis.

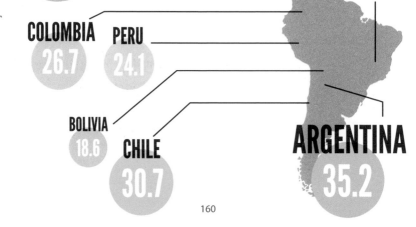

C-SECTION STATISTICS

Percentage of births delivered by caesarean section

IRELAND
26.2

CANADA
26.3

UNITED STATES 30.3

BRAZIL
45.9

37.8 MEXICO

COLOMBIA
26.7

PERU
24.1

BOLIVIA
18.6

CHILE
30.7

ARGENTINA
35.2

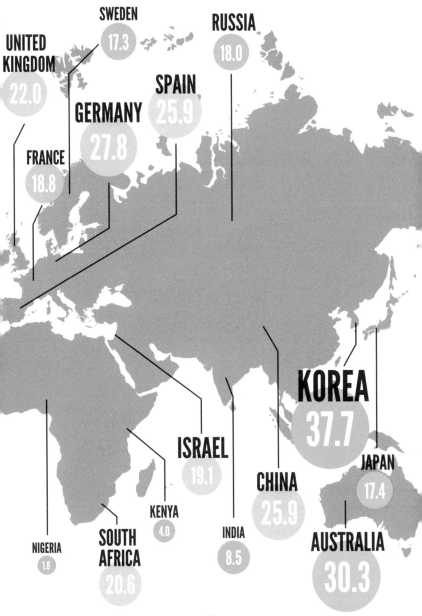

161

PAIN RELIEF: NON-INVASIVE

It's important to know what types of pain relief are available so that you can make informed choices for your birth plan.

Movement

Alternative positions

Gentle massage

Warm shower or bath

Breathing techniques

Warm pack, cool compress or ice pack on painful areas

HYPNOBIRTHING

- This method uses self-hypnosis and visualisation techniques to relax the body and produce enough of the feel-good hormone oxytocin to render pain relief unnecessary

- A course is best taken at 25–30 weeks

- Contractions are renamed 'surges'

- Some studies suggest less intervention is required when hypnobirthing is used. An NHS study in 2012 found the following rates of intervention:

Emergency C-section

General population **15%**

Hypnobirthing mothers **4%**

General population **11%**

Hypnobirthing mothers **8%**

TENS MACHINE

- TENS stands for transcutaneous electrical nerve stimulation

- The machine is a handheld controller connected by leads to four sticky pads placed on your back

- It gives out tiny pulses of electrical energy and produces a tingling sensation on the skin, which can help distract from the pain of contractions, especially during early labour

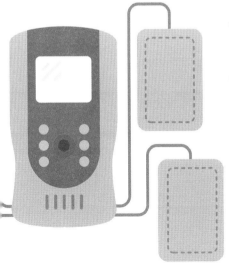

- You can buy these new or hire them for the birth

- TENS is very safe, but its effectiveness is not proven – some mothers may find it provides short-term pain relief, whereas other women may not feel it makes a difference

MEDICAL **PAIN RELIEF**

There are three main types of medical pain relief when you are in labour:

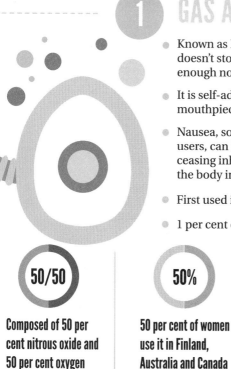

- Known as Entonox, or laughing gas, it doesn't stop the pain, but relaxes you enough not to care as much about it

- It is self-administered via a mouthpiece or facemask

- Nausea, sometimes experienced by users, can be halted by simply ceasing inhalation as the gas leaves the body immediately

- First used in 1934

- 1 per cent of hospitals in the US offer it

50/50

Composed of 50 per cent nitrous oxide and 50 per cent oxygen

50%

50 per cent of women use it in Finland, Australia and Canada

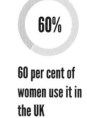

60%

60 per cent of women use it in the UK

Historically, other sedatives such as chloral hydrate (chloroform) and potassium bromide were used. In the 1850s, chloroform was used during the birth of Queen Victoria's last two children.

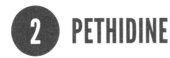

2 PETHIDINE

- An opiate drug, administered via injection into your thigh or buttock

- It works by both relaxing you and offering limited pain relief

- It slows the labour, so it may not be ideal

- Used in the first stage of labour, when the cervix is dilating

- 1 in 3 women use it, but 1 in 3 of these women suffer from nausea and drowsiness

- If the baby is born within 2 hours, it can suffer from lethargy for days later (this can interfere with breastfeeding)

- Less commonly, the drug diamorphine is sometimes used

3 EPIDURAL

- An epidural is a type of local anaesthetic that numbs the pain from the waist down

- It is only administered by a trained anaesthetist when you are in active labour

- Your cervix must be between 5 and 9 cm dilated

- 1 in 100 women have a headache after an epidural

- It may not always be 100 per cent effective: the Obstetric Anaesthetists Association estimates that 1 in 8 women who have an epidural need to use other methods of pain relief

30%

In the UK, 30 per cent of women have an epidural

67%

In the US, 67 per cent of women have an epidural

10 min

It takes around 10 minutes to work

THE FIRST STAGE **OF LABOUR**

Every labour is different, but the average duration of the first stage is around 12 hours – though it may last up to 24 hours or more. There are three stages.

1 Latent Stage

—4 cm—

20 min | 30–45 s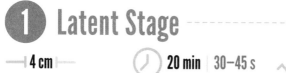

Cervix dilates up to 4 cm

Contractions are roughly 20 minutes apart, lasting 30–45 seconds

Builds in intensity

2 Active Labour

—7 cm—

3–4 min | 45–60 s

Cervix widens from 4 cm to 7 cm, roughly 1 cm per hour

Contractions are 3–4 minutes apart, lasting about 45–60 seconds

May be rather painful and difficult to talk through – breathing exercises, relaxation techniques and pain relief can help

3 Transitional Stage

—7–10 cm—

2–3 min | 60–90 s

Occurs when the cervix is about 7–8 cm dilated, until you are fully dilated (10 cm)

Contractions may be 2–3 minutes apart (or less frequent) but last 60–90 seconds

You will feel the first urge to push

DILATION EXPLAINED

The process by which your body prepares to expel the baby is known as cervical effacement and cervical dilation. Effacement is the thinning of the cervix, whereas dilation is its opening up.

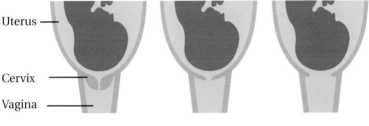

Uterus

Cervix

Vagina

not effaced,
not dilated

fully effaced,
1 cm dilated

fully effaced,
fully dilated

CERVICAL DILATION: A COMPARISON

Coin 2 cm / 0.8 inches

Cracker 4 cm / 1.6 inches

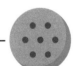

Can 7 cm / 2.75 inches

Doughnut 10 cm / 3.9 inches

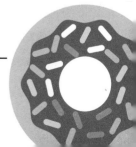

THE SECOND STAGE
OF LABOUR

- Lasts 1–3 hours

- The urge to push has replaced the contractions

- If this stage is too slow, the baby may become distressed

- If it's too quick, there may be tearing

- You must listen to your midwife or doctor to know when to push and how to breathe

- Crowning occurs when the widest part of the baby's head emerges

- Your baby is then finally delivered

The average circumference of a baby's skull is 1 cm larger than the cervix, but luckily the skull is made up of soft and flexible plates of bone with gaps between them, which allow the baby's head to squeeze through the cervix. Eventually, the skull bones will fuse, and the soft spots will close, around a year after birth.

Your uterus will now contract back to the size of a tennis ball

THE THIRD STAGE OF LABOUR

- Lasts 15–60 minutes

- Contractions start again and you may feel the urge to push

- The placenta peels away from the uterus and is delivered

- There are two approaches: active management or physiological care

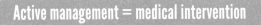

Placenta

Umbilical Cord

Cervix

Vagina

Umbilical Clamp

Active management = medical intervention

1. Use of drugs that contract the uterus

2. Immediate clamping of the umbilical cord (around 20 seconds)

3. The cord is carefully pulled out (controlled cord traction)

Physiological care = intervention occurs only if there is a clinical need

1. Breastfeeding and massage of abdomen are used to contract the uterus

2. Umbilical cord is left to pulse until all the placenta is delivered

3. Placenta is left to be delivered naturally rather than pulled out

 3 out of 10 **midwives use active management**

 More than 9 out of 10 **obstetricians use active management**

COMMON PROBLEMS IN LABOUR

1 BREECH BIRTH

- **The baby will present itself feet or bottom first**
- **A skilful midwife can turn the baby around, or, more often, a caesarean section is performed**

 Around 22 per cent of babies are breech until 28 weeks gestation

 Around 3 per cent are breech at full term

---

2 BACK-TO-BACK LABOUR

- **The baby's spine faces the mother's – leading to a more painful and prolonged birth**
- **Contractions are harder to discern**
- **Often requires an assisted birth**

 15–30 per cent of babies begin labour in this position

 5 per cent of babies are delivered in this position

ASSISTED BIRTH

When?

- If the baby is breech or back-to-back

- If the mother has had a long labour and is finding pushing too hard

- If the baby is becoming distressed

- If the baby is large

- If the mother is overweight, with a BMI of over 30

- If the baby is not low down in the birth canal

Methods

- Caesarean section (see pages 158–9)

- Ventouse, or vacuum-assisted delivery – this suction cup, applied to the baby's head can be used during the second stage of labour, but cannot be used for a breech birth

- Forceps – the use of this surgical instrument to clasp the baby's head carries the risk of certain complications, and has declined significantly in recent decades

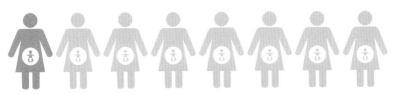

Around 1 in 8 first-time mothers require an assisted birth

Sometimes, in the event of a difficult or elongated labour, an episiotomy is performed. This is a cut in a woman's perineum (the area between the vagina and anus) which allows more room for the baby to pass through. A local anaesthetic is applied to the area, and the cut is usually stitched up within an hour of the birth.

WATER BIRTHS

An increasing number of women are choosing to give birth in a birthing pool. Obstetrician Michel Odent wrote about water birth in the 1970s, but it wasn't until the 1980s that it became more than a niche practice. The Royal College of Obstetricians and Gynaecologists as well as the Royal College of Midwives support the safety of water birth for healthy women with uncomplicated pregnancies.

Things to note

- Water should be no warmer than 37.5°C / 99.5°F
- Being in water may be beneficial during the first stage of labour (when your cervix is at least 5 cm dilated)
- Delivering your baby underwater during the second stage is an experimental procedure with risks involved
- In a hospital setting, you can receive gas and air for pain relief while you are in the pool
- A birth partner can join you in the pool
- You may find an inflatable or waterproof pillow is helpful for resting on

Benefits

- Pain relief due to the warmth of the water
- Helps avoid using other anaesthesia
- Aids relaxation
- Buoyancy makes it easier to change positions
- Speeds up labour

Water birth is usually not suitable if

- Your waters have broken early
- You have a medical condition such as diabetes or epilepsy
- You are very overweight
- You have bled heavily during pregnancy or after birth before
- Your labour is premature (before 37 weeks)
- You need stronger pain relief, e.g. pethidine or an epidural

Possible positions

- Squatting while holding the sides of the pool for support
- Kneeling while leaning forwards on the side of the pool
- Floating on your back with your head supported by a pillow
- Floating on your tummy with your head turned sideways and supported on a pillow
- Sitting with your birth partner behind you

Around 30 per cent of women giving birth in England plan to use a birth pool for coping with pain during labour

Only 6 per cent of women actually give birth in a birth pool

FAMILY **FACTS**

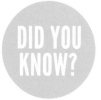

DID YOU KNOW?

According to the Guinness World Records, the woman who gave birth to the largest number of children was the wife of Feodor Vassilyev, a Russian peasant. She lived from 1707 to 1782 and gave birth to:

16 pairs of twins

7 sets of triplets

4 sets of quadruplets

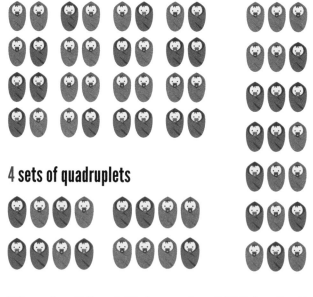

That's 69 children in 27 births!

UK FAMILY SIZE

Families with 1 child **47%**

Families with 2 children **39%**

Families with 3 or more children **14%**

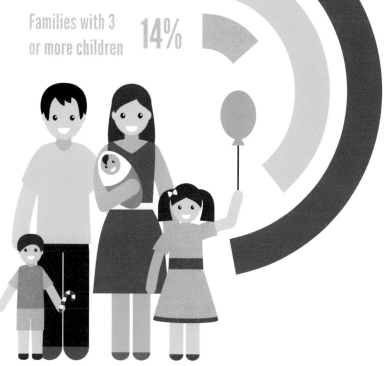

GLOBAL BIRTH STATISTICS

WORLD POPULATION

Estimated world population in 2016

Estimated world population in 2050

7.4 BILLION

9.8 BILLION

350,000 CHILDREN
ARE BORN EACH DAY WORLDWIDE

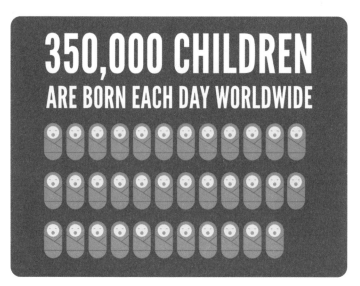

9,230,000 WOMEN GIVE BIRTH EACH MONTH

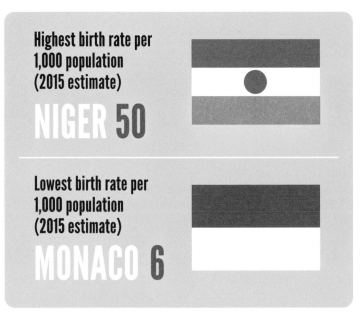

Highest birth rate per 1,000 population (2015 estimate)

NIGER 50

Lowest birth rate per 1,000 population (2015 estimate)

MONACO 6

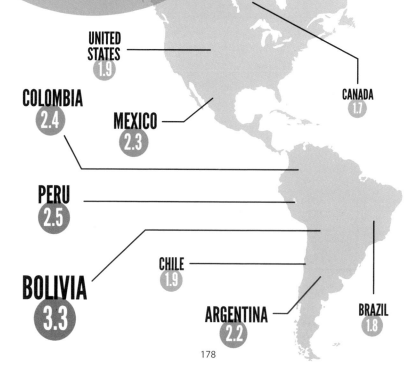

GLOBAL BIRTH STATISTICS

AVERAGE NUMBER OF CHILDREN BORN TO WOMEN OF CHILDBEARING AGE

IRELAND
2.1

UNITED STATES
1.9

CANADA
1.7

COLOMBIA
2.4

MEXICO
2.3

PERU
2.5

BOLIVIA
3.3

CHILE
1.9

ARGENTINA
2.2

BRAZIL
1.8

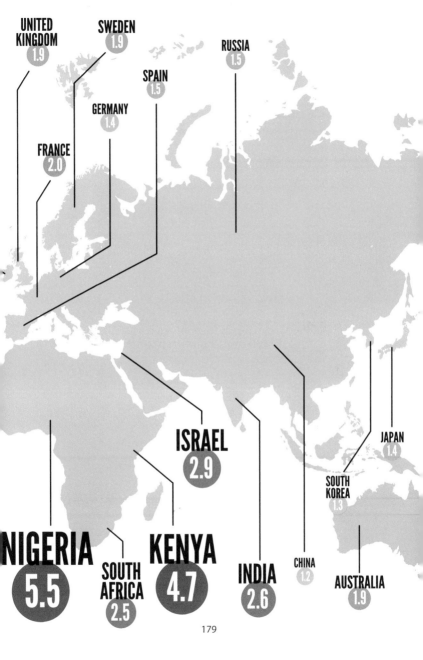

UNITED KINGDOM
1.9

SWEDEN
1.9

RUSSIA
1.5

SPAIN
1.5

GERMANY
1.4

FRANCE
2.0

ISRAEL
2.9

JAPAN
1.4

SOUTH KOREA
1.3

NIGERIA
5.5

SOUTH AFRICA
2.5

KENYA
4.7

INDIA
2.6

CHINA
1.2

AUSTRALIA
1.9

179

MULTIPLE BIRTHS

CHANCES OF MULTIPLE BIRTHS

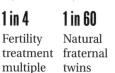

1 in 4
Fertility
treatment
multiple

1 in 60
Natural
fraternal
twins

1 in 250
Natural
identical
twins

1 in 10,000
Natural
triplets

1 in 700,000
Natural
quadruplets

1 in 55,000,000
Natural
quintuplets

FACTORS AFFECTING MULTIPLE BIRTHS

Ethnic background – African people have an increased likelihood of multiple births compared to Asian or Latin American people

Fertility treatment – chances increase when taking fertility medication or undergoing IVF

Maternal family history – chances increase if your mother's family has had multiples in the past

Age – chances increase if the mother is over 35 years old

Pregnancy history – chances increase if a woman has previously had four or more children

If you are a fraternal (non-identical) twin, you have a 1 in 17 chance of having twins yourself.

AVERAGE PREGNANCY LENGTH

Single	38.6 weeks
Twins	35 weeks
Triplets	32 weeks
Quadruplets	30 weeks

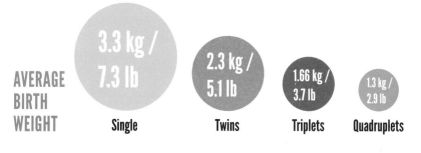

AVERAGE BIRTH WEIGHT

Single	Twins	Triplets	Quadruplets
3.3 kg / 7.3 lb	2.3 kg / 5.1 lb	1.66 kg / 3.7 lb	1.3 kg / 2.9 lb

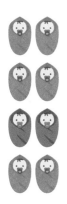

Known in the media as 'Octomom', the American woman Nadya Suleman (born 1975) holds the record for the most number of babies born alive from the same pregnancy: six boys and two girls. They were conceived through IVF treatment and delivered nine weeks prematurely in California on 26 January 2009.

The record for the longest gap between the delivery of twins is 87 days. Amy Ann Elliott was born prematurely in Ireland in June 2012 and her twin sister Kate Marie followed in August 2012.

87 DAYS

GLOSSARY

Amniocentesis – a diagnostic test using a sample of amniotic fluid

Amniotic sac – a membrane that surrounds and protects the foetus

Androgen – a hormone (e.g. testosterone) that produces male sexual characteristics

Artificial insemination – the introduction of semen into the uterus by a means other than sexual intercourse

Blastocyst – an embryo at the stage when it is implanted into the wall of the uterus

Blood sugar level – the amount of glucose in the blood

Braxton Hicks contractions – false contractions where the cervix tightens

Caesarean section – delivery of the baby by surgery

Capillaries – tiny blood vessels which distribute oxygenated blood from the arteries to the tissues of the body and feed deoxygenated blood from the tissues back into the veins

Cervix – the opening of the uterus

Chromosomal disorder – a change in the usual number or structure of chromosomes

Colostrum – a thick, nutrient-rich milk produced by the breasts in the first days after birth

Conception – the creation of a fertilised egg

Contractions – the muscle spasms that tighten and lengthen the uterus during labour

Cramps – small muscle spasms of varying pain levels

Cravings – an urge to consume a particular item of food or drink

CRL – crown–rump length

Deep vein thrombosis – a blood clot that forms in the veins

Diabetes – a disorder where the blood contains high levels of glucose

Diastasis recti – the separation of the stomach muscles during pregnancy

Dilation – the gradual opening of the cervix during labour

Doppler machine – a device that allows the baby's heartbeat to be heard

Down's syndrome – a chromosomal disorder, causing intellectual impairment and physical abnormalities

Early labour – the first stage of labour, when contractions are intermittent and mild

Ectopic pregnancy – the implantation of a fertilised egg outside the uterus, usually in a fallopian tube

Embryo – the developing organism in the first eight weeks after conception

Entonox – otherwise known as 'laughing gas' or 'gas and air' – inhaled to bring about pain relief during childbirth

Enzyme – a substance that serves as a catalyst for biochemical reactions in the body

Epidural – invasive pain relief where the spine is numbed from the waist down

Erectile dysfunction – the inability of the man to achieve or maintain an erection

Established labour – when contractions are regular and close together

Fallopian tube – a tube that runs between the ovary and the uterus

Foetal alcohol syndrome – the condition in a child that results from exposure to alcohol during pregnancy

Foetus – the formal name for the developing baby after the eighth week of pregnancy

Folic acid – a vitamin of the B complex

Forceps – an instrument used to pull out the baby, if needed, during vaginal birth

Gestation – the developmental period inside the uterus between conception and birth

Haemorrhoids – enlarged and swollen veins in the vulval or rectal area, otherwise known as piles

Heartburn – a burning sensation in the chest caused by acid reflux

Hyperemesis gravidarum – severe or prolonged vomiting causing weight loss and dehydration

Hypnobirthing – a hypnotherapy technique which aims to reduce anxiety and pain during childbirth

Incompetent cervix – a weak cervix that may widen during pregnancy, resulting in miscarriage

Induction of labour – starting off labour by artificial means

Insomnia – inability to sleep at night

Instrumental delivery – the use of devices such as forceps to aid the delivery of the baby

IVF – in vitro fertilisation, the process in which the embryo is created outside the womb

Labour – the process of delivering a baby

Ligaments – tissue that connects two bones together

Lightening – when the baby drops into the pelvis, shortly before it is born

Macronutrients – nutrients required by the body in large amounts

Maternity leave – time away from work for the mother, paid for by the employer and/or the government

Micronutrients – vitamins and minerals required by the body in relatively small amounts

Miscarriage – involuntary expulsion of a foetus from the womb when it is too early to develop and survive on its own

Moses basket – a woven wicker basket with a cotton lining, also known as a bassinet

Neural tube defect – genetic defects of the brain or spine in a developing embryo

NICE – National Institute for Health and Care Excellence

NMC – Nursing and Midwifery Council

Non-invasive pain relief – methods by which pain relief is given without surgical intervention

Oesophageal sphincter – muscle fibres connecting the oesophagus and stomach

Oestrogen – a hormone secreted by the ovaries or placenta

Oxytocin – a hormone released by the pituitary gland during labour

Ovulation – the release of an egg from the ovary

Perineum – the area between the vagina and anus

Pessary – a tablet or gel inserted into the vagina in order to stimulate labour

Pethidine – a pain-killing drug

Pica – a craving for non-food items

Placenta – an organ that develops inside a pregnant woman's uterus, supplying nutrients and oxygen to the foetus through the umbilical cord

Placental abruption – condition where the placenta becomes separated from the uterine wall

Placenta praevia – condition where the placenta partially or completely covers the cervix

Polycystic ovary syndrome – a hormonal condition which disrupts regular ovulation and affects fertility

Postnatal – the first month after birth

Pre-eclampsia – a late-pregnancy condition characterised by high blood pressure

Premature labour – any labour which begins before 37 weeks of pregnancy

Progesterone – a hormone that stimulates the uterus to prepare for pregnancy

Prostaglandin – a substance that has hormone-like effects, notably the promotion of uterine contractions

Quad screen blood test – otherwise known as the quadruple marker test – used to gauge the likelihood of any complications or birth defects

RCOG – Royal College of Obstetricians and Gynaecologists

RCM – Royal College of Midwives

Relaxin – the hormone that loosens the ligaments in preparation for labour

Restless leg syndrome – a nervous system disorder that results in a constant desire to move the legs

Rubella – a contagious virus that can lead to birth defects if contracted when pregnant

Rupture of membranes – when the waters (amniotic fluid) break during labour

SIDS – sudden infant death syndrome

SPD – symphysis pubis dysfunction, pelvic joint pain during pregnancy or childbirth

Sperm count – the number of spermatozoa present in each ejaculation

Spina bifida – when the neural tube that becomes the spine and brain fails to close properly at the embryonic stage of pregnancy

STI – sexually transmitted infection

Stillbirth – the birth of a dead foetus

Stress incontinence – involuntary urination when pressure in the body increases, such as when coughing

Syntocinon – synthetic oxytocin

TENS – a type of pain relief that uses electrical nerve stimulation

Testosterone – a hormone that ensures the development of male sexual characteristics

Toxoplasmosis – a parasitic disease transmitted through soil, cat faeces, or undercooked meat; it is dangerous to unborn children

Trimester – a period of three months

Ultrasound scan – a method of viewing the baby within the abdomen, using sound waves

Uterus – the womb

Vaginal birth – the natural delivery of a baby

Ventouse – the delivery of a baby via the vagina with the assistance of a suction cup attached to the baby's head

Vulva – the external opening of the female sexual organs

NOTE ON SOURCES

The infographics and recommendations in this book have been created using data from a range of sources. While care has been taken to ensure that this information is accurate and up to date, the author and publisher cannot accept responsibility for any inaccuracies in data collected and analysed by other organisations. In general, if global data is not available, or if consensus on certain topics does not exist, the information given in this book relates to the United Kingdom and follows the recommendations of the National Health Service. As statistics and guidance on pregnancy are liable to change over time, professional advice should be sought in case of any doubt. The following sources of information have been consulted in the preparation of this book:

- World Health Organization (who.int)
- Office for National Statistics (www.ons.gov.uk)
- NHS Choices (www.nhs.uk)
- National Institute for Health and Care Excellence (www.nice.org.uk)
- Human Fertilisation and Embryology Authority (www.hfea.gov.uk)
- Equality and Human Rights Commission (www.equalityhumanrights.com)
- Population Matters (www.populationmatters.org)
- World Family Map (www.worldfamilymap.ifstudies.org)
- Guinness World Records (www.guinnessworldrecords.com)

IMAGE CREDITS

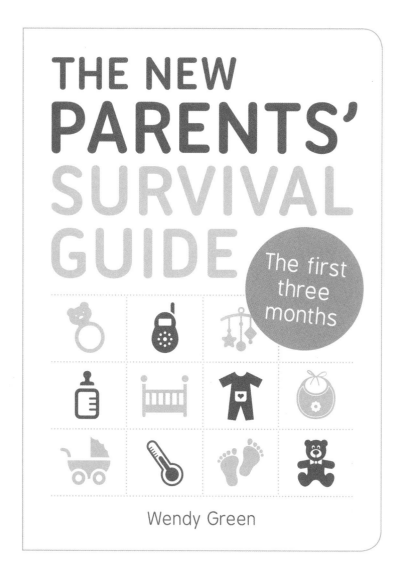

THE NEW PARENTS' SURVIVAL GUIDE

The first three months

Wendy Green

THE NEW PARENTS' SURVIVAL GUIDE

Wendy Green

£7.99
Paperback
ISBN: 978 1 84953 715 5

Everything you need to know to guide you through your baby's first three months and beyond!

No matter how much you long for and plan for a baby, no one is quite prepared for the impact their new arrival has on their life. This book recognises that no one has a textbook-perfect baby and lets you in on what you can REALLY expect in the first three months. *The New Parents' Survival Guide* is packed with practical advice and simple tips on how to deal with common problems you are likely to encounter, including how to:

- Care for your newborn
- Solve the breast versus bottle dilemma
- Overcome breastfeeding woes
- Calm your crying baby
- Solve sleep issues
- Manage minor ailments
- Take good care of yourself

Have you enjoyed this book?
If so, why not write a review on your favourite website?

If you're interested in finding out more about our books,
find us on Facebook at Summersdale Publishers and
follow us on Twitter at @Summersdale.

Thanks very much for buying this Summersdale book.

www.summersdale.com